5 Fast Flat Belly Facts

Unlock the Secrets to a Slimmer, Healthier You

Dr. Amanda Borre, D.C.

of the information contained within this document, including, but not limited to, errors, omissions, or inaccuracies.

Table of Contents

Introduction

A flat tummy: The secret weapon to a healthy life.
–Best Slogans, n.d.

Ever since I came across this phrase, I have not been able to stop thinking about how powerful it is! Time and again, we have been told how our body weight affects our overall health. An excessive increase or decrease in weight is typically an alarming indication of various underlying health conditions. Yet, throughout the decades, society's conception of aesthetics has depended a lot on a person's weight and size. From beauty pageants to the movies, slim people are portrayed as appealing and beautiful. The good news is that many of these superficial beauty standards all across the globe are shifting, and I'm delighted to live in an era where individuals have started focusing on their uniqueness, self-love, and self-expression. This is a source of hope for me and undoubtedly for many others like me.

However, from a medical point of view, we cannot deny that gaining too much weight can lead to a myriad of health issues. Obesity and the accumulation of visceral fat—or belly fat—are some of the leading causes of serious health conditions, such as cardiovascular diseases, high blood pressure, certain cancers, stroke, gallstones, diabetes, and many more. So, while being overweight or having excessive fat density is not necessarily an aesthetic concern, it should not be neglected because it adds to the risk factors for your health. Maintaining a healthy weight is vital to preventing and controlling several conditions and diseases.

You've probably heard that as you get older, you are more likely to gain weight or add inches around your belly and other portions of your body. Your metabolism—which is mostly in charge of managing your body's weight—functions significantly differently or, rather, a bit slower as you get older. And while this is true, you shouldn't use it as an excuse to give up on your efforts to get healthy. Get after it! You *can* make a change!

Given our hectic lifestyles, the hustle and bustle of daily life, and the jobs and commitments that hang over us all, it makes sense that you might feel like you don't have enough time to pause and evaluate your overall well-being. However, these conditions are an inevitable aspect of life, and we can't downplay the significance of maintaining good health and fitness in the light of advancing years and stressful situations. Your health should always be a priority—no matter what.

According to research, "Most of the world's population live in countries where overweight and obesity kill more people than underweight" (World Health Organization, 2021). Obesity and being overweight are conditions where there is an overabundance of fat in the body, which can cause severe health damage. So, your waistline has a lot to do with your overall health, and a lot of us are in trouble. I say we turn these statistics around.

Doctors emphasize the fact that the fat around the belly is the most dangerous of all types of fat. This is because the accumulation of such fat starts in the abdominal region and gradually spreads into other organs (Lemos, 2020).

Fat content is always present in the human body. However, the problem arises when there is an imbalance in the amount and type of fat deposit. For instance, the fat that lies immediately under your skin is called subcutaneous fat. You can feel this type of fat by pinching your skin. Visceral fat, on the other hand, is found in your intestines and stomach areas. Visceral fat is mostly responsible for the formation of various ailments in your body.

Research also shows that larger waist size can be a huge concern—for women, more than 35 inches, and for men, more than 40 inches (Wade, 2015). This is a prime reason why it's necessary to shed extra fat around the belly to stay fit in the long run.

Abdominal obesity is strongly linked to various health conditions. So, losing or, rather, reaching a healthy weight and size can have tremendous advantages to your holistic health. Here are some of the most important reasons why having a healthy body and a flat tummy is so crucial for everyone, regardless of age or gender:

- A healthy BMI and a flatter tummy can help prevent many diseases. Abdominal obesity is associated with a high risk of cardiovascular diseases, hypertension, type 2 diabetes, asthma, sleep apnea, Alzheimer's disease, and insulin resistance. Also, with an increase in the waist and hip ratio, there is a greater chance of developing conditions such as blood lipid disorders, metabolic syndrome, and various other physical ailments (Westphal, 2008).

- The size of your waist can also be related to knee osteoarthritis. Obese people are more likely to experience aches, which can have a severe impact on their flexibility and mobility. A flatter tummy can make you feel healthier and also help you stay active and swift for a longer time. Visceral fat plays a strong role in affecting your body's functioning, and by reducing it, you can stay fit and healthy. Simply put, visceral fat helps produce cytokines, an inflammatory chemical, which can cause inflammation and lead to autoimmune and neurodegenerative diseases (Wade, 2015).

- Health is not only about your physical condition; it is also about your mental state. Research shows that excessive fat in the abdomen can adversely affect cognitive functions (Dolan, 2023). By keeping a check on the growing fat around your midsection and your overall weight, you can help prevent many diseases caused by lifestyle issues. Obesity can also play a major role in how you operate in your day-to-day life. From self-esteem issues and difficulty conducting regular activities to developing life-threatening diseases, your growing weight and size can cause serious disruptions to your normal routine. Your physical *and* mental health can benefit from working toward a more fit and healthy life.

I think you'll agree with me when I say that weight gain is tricky to understand. For example, you might be eating healthy and working out daily, but you simply cannot lose any weight. Contrary to popular belief, consuming more food is not the only thing that results in weight gain. In fact, weight gain can result from a variety of factors. Hormonal imbalance, sugar and sodium consumption, medications, certain health conditions, and not having a well-rounded diet can lead to a higher accumulation of fat and an increase in your overall weight.

Let me share an interesting thing I recently came across while scrolling through a social media page. Edna, a middle-aged, plus-sized woman, lost 20 pounds in only a couple of weeks. When I came across this video, I started watching, feeling curious, interested, and quite inspired until toward the end, she pulled out a package of some "magic" tea bags and showed it to the viewers. As a wellness and health fanatic, I was taken aback when I heard her say she lost a considerable amount of body fat and dramatically reduced her weight by simply sipping the "tea" for a month and doing nothing more! By the time I could fully understand that this was a commercial that only looked like a person genuinely telling her story, I had already started to feel uneasy about how the weight-loss industry has taken the world by storm—in quite an adverse way!

I find it unfortunate that we live in an age when there is nearly unlimited access to information, but it is a challenge to figure out what is genuine and what is not. These days, the market is mostly digitized and relies on marketing techniques that only look real to customers. In the case of Edna, I was hooked on the video and was interested right until the end, when I figured out what she "did" to make her weight vanish in only a few days. And while the medical professional in me found it appalling and unrealistic, I cannot deny that I was watching the video very attentively. This type of marketing is part of the real problem and can be very dangerous in the long term. I realized that there must be millions like me watching the video, and many of them were probably buying what she was selling!

That's how business works, right? But, seriously, I am not up for it! It was then that I decided to make a real effort to bring the truth to people trying to lose weight. I became determined to help them achieve their goals by guiding them in the most practical and healthiest way possible. From a health and medical point of view, I fully understand the disadvantages of gaining weight (and more so, visceral fat). Your health is important, so what you use on and in your body has to be "marked safe" before using it—because even a small glitch can make you suffer.

Just like a parent strives to give the best possible advice and the finest quality food to their children, please realize that you have to be equally wary about your own health and fitness. If weight loss and shedding a few inches from your belly is your goal, then your priority should also be turning to the most authentic ways to get there. Don't depend on fad diets and tricks that seldom work and also have probable side effects. Join me on this journey where we dig into the treasure trove of knowledge that will help you gain an understanding of how your body operates.

We all have ideas about how we can lose weight, but there are specific aspects we need to look into further. First, it is essential to comprehend the root causes of weight gain. Yes, every time you look in the mirror and see a slight double chin peeking out or pull on a pair of jeans that suddenly seem a little too tight, such can be your body's way of telling you that you are weighing in a bit more than usual. And while the physical aspects of weight issues are visible, we also need to address the unseen psychological aspects.

Unfortunately, societal pressures and stereotypical judgments based on a person's weight often outweigh (pun intended) many other beautiful features they possess. Many people today—maybe even you!—still measure their worth through the weight on a scale. Let me set this straight: Your weight does not define you! My whole point is to make you understand that losing weight should never be about how others perceive you or how much you want them to approve of you. It has to be with only one perspective—and that is to improve your health and lead a long, vital life.

If you think about it, when you were younger, you could run up the stairs and not pant. With age or with a few extra pounds, it could get difficult to even take the stairs up to the second floor, let alone run! This is what fitness is about; the stubborn weight or a growing belly can make you feel exhausted and unwell and even dwindle your self-esteem at times. While some people recognize these problems and work on them right away, others might feel like they can't do anything due to a lack of time, focus, or even a sense of guilt about taking care of themselves. Taking a few minutes each day to work on yourself is not much to ask for; but I also understand that for many, it can be a huge challenge.

One solution to such situations is to understand your health inside and out and how it relates to your holistic well-being. You do not have to have a fancy gym membership or buy products that promise to trim your waist. All you have to do is stay with me until the end of this book, understand how our body works, and learn how you can use it to your benefit. We will talk about the top five ways to keep your weight, body fat, and, most importantly, your general well-being in the best shape possible. Through years of meticulous study and research, I have come up with interesting ways to understand why having a flat tummy is important and how you can achieve it by simply following a few methods.

You chose this book because something inside makes you think you need motivation and—most importantly—some guidance to achieve a certain fitness level demonstrated by a flatter stomach. Bravo for the decision you made to take a step forward and learn ways to feel and look better. You are already taking action by seeking help and reading to learn more. Here are a few areas you will have a better understanding of by the time you finish reading this book:

- **Your health matters.** This book is carefully crafted to help you understand how important your health is and how everything else revolves around it. It will boost your confidence as you read about every little detail of how your body works, inside and out. The more you get into the intricacies of your physical and mental health, you will be able to incorporate that knowledge into your weight loss and waist-reduction process.

- **Your food matters.** Most of the time, we think that losing weight and staying fit is about not eating as much, but with the help of the various topics covered in this book, you will get a clear picture of how food can affect your overall health. I'll cover the foods that can be helpful and the foods that can put you in danger to help you make smart and careful choices.

At the end of the day, this is how you can rediscover happiness with yourself. By revitalizing your inner strength and working things through intelligently, you'll be able to enjoy a fresh outlook and a newfound zeal.

The adage "Prevention is better than cure" sums up how taking care of your health at the right time can help you stay in good spirits and health for the rest of your life, and starting your fitness journey is not limited to a certain age, gender, or body type. Whatever stage of life you are in, taking steps to get healthy again is important. It doesn't matter if you are a student who feels overweight and uneasy, you are one of the busiest people around, you have recently recovered from a medical condition, or you are retired. All it takes to significantly enhance your quality of life is the will to work on yourself and the effort to make a few slight modifications to the way you live. In no time, you will feel the difference and come to meet the healthier version of yourself. There is no time like the present—so let's get started!

Chapter 1:

Sodium Sensitivity

On certain days, when you wake up in the morning, you may notice that your face feels puffier than usual. Well, in some cases, you can blame the delicious food you consumed the previous day. In a situation like this, you will notice that no amount of lymphatic drainage massages or gua sha can come to the rescue. Food with a high sodium content can be one of the biggest causes of water retention in your body, especially in your stomach.

As a teenager, I remember my brother and I poured salt into my mom's water glass on a vacation to the rodeo. She was so swollen, she couldn't get her boots off! We thought we were *hilarious*. Her? Not so much. Sodium sensitivity is real and can adversely affect your health in many ways.

Every time sodium is mentioned, most people tend to think about salt. Though not wrong, there is a slight difference in salt and sodium, which is quite interesting to understand. Sodium is a dietary mineral that is required for muscle and nerve functions and to balance the body's fluids and minerals. Salt, on the other hand, contains 40% sodium and 60% chloride (Harvard School of Public Health, 2019). Salt is also known as sodium chloride for this reason. We season our meals with table salt, which is mostly composed of sodium chloride. Simply put, sodium is present in salt.

In numerous cases, sodium sensitivity is referred to as salt sensitivity, which is a change in health condition mainly caused by an increase or decrease in sodium intake. Blood pressure is one of the major areas that is highly affected by sodium sensitivity issues. This can further lead to many medical complications and conditions, like hypertension, cardiovascular diseases, and even stroke. Understanding the role of sodium in your health and everything related to it can be one of the best ways to keep track of your nutrition and health conditions, as well as keep your waist trim.

Understanding Sodium Intake

The U.S. Food and Drug Administration (FDA) has made huge efforts to curb the excessive sodium contained in mostly packaged and processed foods. We consume about 70% of the sodium in our diets through packaged food. This is one of the reasons why keeping track of what you eat and the nutritional content of packaged food is very important (FDA, 2020). And while imagining a saltless diet can seem pretty boring, it is also true that the excessive sodium present in salt can be harmful. So, understanding sodium intake is very important for your health.

Recommended Daily Allowance

The average American consumes about 3,400 milligrams (mg) of sodium per day, which is more than double the federal recommendation (CDC, 2019). The American Heart Association recommends around 1,500 mg of sodium daily. However, a more practical goal is to not consume more than 2,300 mg of sodium each day (Creekside Family Practice, n.d.).

Sources of Hidden Sodium

Many times, people begin a low-sodium diet for medical and weight-loss reasons. They avoid known sodium, but despite their best efforts, they continue to experience concerns with bloating, water retention, and high blood pressure. Unknown sources of salt in your diet may also be a major contributing factor.

If you have experienced this, you might want to food journal to pinpoint potential causes. For instance, countless food items have sodium, which may not be easy to track unless you are journaling to look back at symptoms versus food intake. Here are a few food items that are some of the sneakiest places where sodium hides:

- sauces, like soy, oyster, Worcestershire, pasta, etc.

- canned foods, like soups, stews, and other food items

- seasoning, condiments, bouillon, ready-made pastes, meat tenderizers, and dressings for food and salads

- frozen meals with sauces and gravy

- processed and packaged food, like salted chips, popcorn, pretzels, crackers, pork rinds, biscuits, noodles, pasta, vegetables, sausages, nuggets, cereals, etc.

- cured, canned, and smoked meat and fish

- different types of cheese and deli meats

- ready-made mixes like pudding, cakes, etc.

- egg whites and cottage cheese (These are the two that surprised me most!)

Apart from these sneaky sodium items, you can even find sodium in small traces in several medicines. Consulting your medical practitioner regarding any of your medical conditions and medications can be a good way to understand what you are consuming.

Reading the back of nutrition labels is a great habit to get into for many reasons. Many times, items that are termed "low-calorie" or "low-sodium" may trick you into believing that there is very little to no sodium at all. However, it is always a good idea to be aware of what you are consuming by checking the details and labels of food products carefully.

Effects of Excessive Sodium

Have you recently experienced feeling excessively thirsty and bloated? This could be one or more of the symptoms of consuming excessive sodium! As we've already seen, there are countless types of food sources that might contain sodium, so keeping a check on the total amount in all the foods you are consuming regularly can be difficult.

If sodium is not taken in moderation or smaller amounts, this might result in a number of health issues as well. Here are some of the ways excessive sodium can affect you if you don't take control:

Water Retention and Bloating

Too much sodium can cause swelling in various parts of the body, mostly in the ankles, feet, legs, face, hands, and stomach. This condition is also known as edema, and it can also be influenced by many underlying health conditions that cause the tissues to accumulate more fluid than needed.

Studies have shown how an increase in sodium intake can cause bloating. According to the National Library of Medical Science, reducing sodium is a crucial dietary intervention that can help reduce bloating and other related symptoms (Peng et al., 2019).

There are days when you feel heavier than usual and particularly not at your best. The chances are you are facing some water retention issues in your system. Here are some signs and symptoms that could hint at this condition:

- swollen parts of the body, like a puffy face and feet

- bloating in the stomach and abdomen

- fluctuation in weight, like sudden weight gain in only a few days

- reduced flexibility and stiff feeling in the joints

- visible indent forming when pressing on the swollen areas of the body

- body aches

Aside from sodium, there are many reasons why you might retain water, including long periods of traveling on flights, prolonged sitting or standing, health conditions, medications, pregnancy, menstruation, hormonal fluctuations, liver and kidney issues, etc.

Fluid retention can be classified into two categories: generalized edema and localized edema. In the first case, the entire body gets swollen, and in the second case, only specific body parts get swollen. As already mentioned, there could be many reasons for this, but a very common cause of mild water retention is excessive consumption of sodium or salt (Better Health Channel, 2012).

Regardless of what type of water retention you may be facing, it is very important to understand the real diagnosis or cause of the condition. Proper consultation with a doctor, physical tests, and investigating medical history are crucial to help prevent or cure any medical condition in the long run.

Here are a few strategies to help you significantly reduce water retention:

- **Swap out high-sodium foods:** Replace sodium-laden food sources with low-sodium foods or alternatives. Table salt is a source of sodium, but the hidden sodium content in many foods can be problematic. Almost 75% of the sodium consumed by most people comes not from cooking salt but from other unnoticed sources of food. Checking the quality and content of all food items before consumption is the best way to control sodium intake (Smith, 2023).

- **Drink more water:** Dehydration can cause the body to retain more fluid in the system, causing water retention issues. Drinking enough water is the best way to prevent this condition. It can also help flush toxins and bacteria from your bladder; prevent digestive issues; regulate blood pressure and body temperature; protect various organs, tissues, and joints; and regulate sodium or electrolyte balance in your system (Harvard Health Publishing, 2020). I recommend drinking half your body weight in ounces per day, with a tad more on super sweaty days.

In addition to these techniques, living a healthy lifestyle that includes eating clean and exercising regularly can enhance the body's blood circulation, which in turn can help the lymphatic drainage process and the body's ability to expel toxins.

Impact on Blood Pressure

The World Health Organization (WHO) recommends keeping a count on sodium intake because of its effect on blood pressure. As per the WHO's recommendation, reducing sodium intake to less than 2 grams a day, which is almost 5 grams of salt per day, for all adults will prevent hypertension, cardiovascular diseases, coronary heart diseases, and even stroke (World Health Organization, 2012).

An increase in blood pressure can impact your health in many ways. In many cases, it goes back to the point of salt sensitivity. For instance, sodium intake can impact a person's blood pressure but not affect another's at all. Age, weight, and, in many cases, race also play a significant role in salt-sensitivity issues (Cleveland Clinic, 2017).

An increase in blood pressure typically comes with certain signs and warnings. It is critical to comprehend a few symptoms of high blood pressure to prevent any problems. So, here are some symptoms you should be aware of:

- severe headaches

- exhaustion

- vision problems

- difficulty breathing

- irregular heart rhythm

- blood in the urine or nosebleed

- pounding sensation in the chest, ears, and neck

Apart from these signs, some people can get seizures, sweating, nervousness, blood spots in the eyes, sleeping issues, and feelings of confusion as well. Fluctuations in blood pressure can cause serious health issues, so keeping a blood pressure monitor at home or measuring your pressure often is a good idea if you are concerned (Sachdev, 2023).

According to the National Library of Medicine, hypertension can most affect organs such as the kidneys, heart, and brain. These are the target organs that are more likely to be damaged in cases of uncontrolled blood pressure (Mensah et al., 2002).

Let's look at a few ways rising blood pressure or hypertension can damage your health (Mayo Clinic, 2022):

Heart

High blood pressure can lead to several types of cardiovascular issues. Conditions such as an enlarged left heart, coronary artery disease, and even heart failure are very common for people suffering from long-term hypertension. The blood supply to the heart gets affected by the blood pressure because arteries get damaged from the pressure that is applied to supply blood to the heart. Similarly, when the heart pumps very fast to meet the circulation of blood in the body, it causes an enlarged left heart. Moreover, hypertension can cause so much stress on the heart that it fails to work, causing severe health conditions and even death.

Kidneys

Blood vessels and those connected to the kidneys can be damaged because of hypertension. For the kidneys to function and filter waste from the body, it is imperative to have healthy blood vessels. Kidney scarring, also known as glomerulosclerosis, leading to kidney failure, is one of the conditions that a rise in blood pressure can aggravate. In such cases, the blood vessels that connect to and are in the kidneys get so damaged that they start preventing the kidneys from filtering the toxins from the body, which can even lead to kidney failure.

Brain

The body, especially the brain, depends heavily on healthy blood circulation. A dysfunctional blood supply to the brain can lead to a variety of disorders, including transient ischemic attack (TIA), dementia, and stroke. TIA is also referred to as a ministroke. It is caused by high blood pressure due to blood clots and disruption of the supply of blood to the brain. TIA is a small stroke; however, it may also be a sign of a more serious or larger stroke. When the brain is deprived of nutrients and oxygen, the brain cells get depleted. Hypertension can cause ruptures or leaks in the blood vessels, which can further lead to stroke. Apart from these conditions, mild cognitive impairment and dementia are also conditions that can result from prolonged hypertension issues.

Eyes

The blood vessels that connect to the eyes can get damaged due to hypertension. High blood pressure can cause conditions like retinopathy, optic neuropathy, and choroidopathy. Retinopathy can cause the eyes to bleed, blur the vision, and, in many cases, also cause the eyes to lose vision. Choroidopathy is a condition where there is fluid accumulation under the retina, which can cause distorted vision and loss of vision. Optic neuropathy refers to nerve damage that is caused by hypertension; blood circulation gets blocked, which further damages the optic nerve, causing bleeding and loss of vision as well. High blood pressure can also cause other conditions such as glaucoma, retinal vein occlusion, hemorrhages, narrowing of blood vessels, and stroke risk.

High blood pressure is a risk factor for numerous health problems, and it is considered to be extremely risky to have hypertension when pregnant or with an underlying medical condition, like diabetes. From memory to vision, almost every aspect of the body and mind can be harmed if hypertension is not kept in check regularly.

Personal Anecdote

Left turn here and unrelated to blood pressure per se, but health and heart related for sure: One surprising thing I heard recently was about a colleague of my husband. He was boarding a flight and noticed that his legs were unusually fatigued from walking through the airport. He later felt a heaviness in his chest and a pain in his arm. Now, the symptoms of chest pain and arm pain are total red flags we all have heard about, but the heaviness in his legs was new. He listened to his body, left the airport, and headed for the Emergency Room. He had a 70% blockage in the "widow maker," a common vessel to be occluded and cause sudden death. He was able to get a stint put in and lived to tell the tale. He cautioned my husband and their fellow desk jockey colleagues to be aware of that symptom that likely saved his life, so I'm passing it along here too.

Strategies for Managing Sodium Intake

One of my very dear friends would wake up every morning looking like she was three months pregnant. I would wonder how that could be true because I would be with her most of the time, and she was a very light eater. Every morning before heading off to work, she would look at the mirror and, with her tiny fingers, press on her stomach, and it would look and feel swollen. She would lose her confidence for the entire day by starting the day in a bad mood!

This continued for a long time until we thought of investigating what she had been consuming the previous day and what was making her feel like this. We found out that the food she was eating almost every evening, though lower in calories, was pretty high in salt content. She was an ardent lover of soups, so she would use the bouillon powder and soup mixture to prepare her dinner soup, and that was, in fact, causing the extreme bloating every day!

As we know, sodium can be one of the culprits for many of your health conditions. From water retention issues to managing your blood pressure, what you eat and drink plays a significant role. Controlling your salt intake can be a great step toward improving your health.

Here are a few strategies that could help you manage your sodium intake:

Pink Himalayan Salt

According to Healthy Human Life in an article published in Sept 2023, updated October 2023, Pink Himalayan salt has many benefits (*Incredible Benefits of Himalayan Salt*, 2023):

Nutritional Benefits

- For centuries, people who live in "Blue Zones" have relied on a Mediterranean diet. Sea salt is a central part of the Mediterranean way of eating that studies show leads to longevity. Himalayan salt's rich mineral content can help your body detoxify.

- Himalayan salt contains more than 80 minerals and elements, including potassium, iron, and calcium. All of these minerals aid our body's natural detoxification process and promote the removal of bacteria. It contains less sodium than processed table salt and lowers blood pressure. Table salt is highly processed and contains fewer minerals and more sodium than Himalayan salt does. When you swap table salt for Himalayan salt, your body has an easier time processing it because it doesn't require as much water to clear out the excess sodium as it would have if you had consumed table salt.

- To boot, Himalayan salt is naturally rich in iodine, which food companies add artificially to table salt after processing. The natural iodine in Himalayan salt is very effective at helping your body create an electrolyte balance, helping your intestines absorb nutrients, and lowering blood pressure. Contrary to what most people believe, Himalayan salt can aid hydration. Want a great post-workout hack? Drink some Himalayan salt and lemon water.

- The average adult body is approximately 65% water. If we don't drink the 64 ounces or so of water we all need a day (as most of us don't!), our bodies feel it. If the body's water content drops by as little as 2%, we will feel fatigued. How can Himalayan salt and lemon water help? The same way popular sports drinks do. Essentially, when we sweat or work out, we lose minerals or electrolytes. Drinking water with a pinch of mineral-rich Himalayan salt after a workout can help you regain them and, in turn, boost your energy and hydration.

- Himalayan salt's rich mineral content helps balance the body's pH levels. When your pH levels are balanced, your body has better immunity and is better able to process and digest food.

- Do you tend to wake up at 3 a.m.? There's a reason why! This is one of the most common times of night for people to wake up and struggle with sleep, and it can be linked to salt intake. Between 2 a.m. and 4 a.m., biochemical reactions can occur because of high levels of stress hormones that flush through your system and cause sleep disturbances or interrupt your ability to stay asleep. Studies show that low-sodium diets cause blood volume to decrease in the sympathetic nervous system, which, in turn, activates adrenaline and the fight-or-flight response. For a great night's sleep, try mixing some raw honey with a pinch of Himalayan salt and either eat it straight or dissolve it in a cup of tea.

Therapeutic Benefits

- Himalayan salt isn't just for eating! Combine Himalayan salt with coconut oil to exfoliate dry, winter skin, or use a pink Himalayan salt lamp to purify your air.

- Holistic medical practitioners tout Himalayan salt lamps for their ability to purify indoor air, reduce allergies, and improve your overall well-being. Salt is naturally hygroscopic, which means that it attracts water to its surface. The light from the Himalayan lamp causes the water absorbed by it to evaporate quickly. So, although there are few studies on Himalayan salt lamps, it makes sense that they would help with mold reduction and allergies.

- A nightstand set with salt (the lamp kind!) is an easy way to improve your mood and well-being. In addition to purifying the air, the glow of Himalayan salt lamps is a great antithesis to the digital light we often look at just before we go to sleep. A growing body of research shows that exposure to "blue light"—the kind that radiates from our phones, computers, and tablets— actually winds us *up* as we are trying to wind *down*.

- Himalayan salt lamps naturally produce a soft, warm glow that is similar to what a candle or campfire would produce. They're the perfect night-lights for your or your kids' rooms.

- Additionally, Himalayan salt lamps produce a small amount of negative ions—odorless, tasteless molecules found in abundance in natural environments, such as mountains and beaches. Some studies suggest that these ions can boost serotonin and alleviate symptoms of depression.

- You can also get rid of that dry winter skin with a homemade Himalayan salt exfoliator. Himalayan salt makes a great natural exfoliator. Mix the salt crystals with olive oil or coconut oil and use it with a warm washcloth or in a warm bath for smoother, softer skin.

- Salt and mineral baths are a great way to relieve sore or cramped muscles. So, soothe sore muscles with a Himalayan salt bath. Mineral baths make it easy for your body to absorb the magnesium and other trace minerals in the salt, which can fortify bones and connective tissue that may be contributing to soreness.

Challenge!

Tomorrow morning, why not add a pinch of Himalayan salt to your water? Squeeze some lemon in it for added nutrients and bring it with you when you're on the go.

Reading Labels and Making Informed Choices

They may seem small, but the impact of even minor positive changes can have a huge impact on your health. By adopting certain modifications in your lifestyle and habits, you can stay healthy and keep yourself safe from many medical challenges now and in the future.

I get it. Measuring your food and the sodium in it every single day can be a grueling task, especially if you have a hectic schedule. However, in America, people tend to consume much more sodium than the recommended amount. This is one of the reasons why the U.S. Food and Drug Administration (FDA) is leaving no stone unturned in its efforts to curb sodium consumption.

While it may seem tedious, reading nutritional facts labels whenever you buy a food item and making informed choices about what you consume and in what portions can help you manage your health (U.S. Food and Drug Administration, 2021).

To help simplify, here are two things to focus on when you read nutritional facts labels:

1. **Per Serving:** Read the Per Serving quantity and guidelines before consuming the food. For instance, most items have a quantity based on one serving. Make sure to read and understand how much is recommended.

2. **Daily Value:** It's important to understand the proper dosage of any item you consume, especially sodium. Keep a note of the percentage of sodium present and monitor how much you are consuming.

Making healthy choices is key to leading a healthy life, but reading and understanding labels can be tricky. Here are some easy tips to help you understand them, according to the FDA (2020):

- If the label of the food product says "salt or sodium free," then that means it has less than 5 mg of sodium per serving.

- "Very low sodium" means less than 35 mg of sodium per serving.

- "Low sodium" means less than 140 mg of sodium per saving.

- "Reduced sodium" means that the product contains 25% less sodium than in its original version.

- "Light in sodium" or "lightly salted" means that the product contains 50% less sodium than in the original state.

- "No salt added" or "unsalted" means that the product may not necessarily be unsalted. It simply means that no salt was added during the processing of the product.

Reading labels helps, but one of the best methods to keep track of how much sodium you consume regularly is to cook and prepare your own food!

Cooking Tips for Reducing Sodium

Let's look at some easy ways to reduce sodium intake when cooking at home:

- **Read the label:** Always check the nutritional labels of the products you buy. A major amount of sodium you consume regularly is found in packaged food items used for cooking and enhancing flavor. Ensure that you read the correct serving size and the sodium content to be sure of how much to use.

- **Remember: Fresh is best:** Buy fresh food instead of processed and frozen food options. Ensure that you check the label to see if brine water has been added to preserve the meat or other products. Opt for local and seasonal fruits and vegetables so you can prepare your food with items that are less contaminated and not grown with extra chemicals and fertilizers. Many long-preserved items contain coatings of preservatives used to keep them fresh for a long time, which is one of the main reasons to choose seasonal food items. Also, shopping for fresh goods will benefit your local farmers and businesses as well!

- **Put down the salt shaker:** Sprinkling extra salt on food while eating is more of a habit than a need and can be harmful in many ways. Avoid keeping table salt on the dining table or even on the counter to prevent the temptation to add more to your food. While cooking, keep the salt level as low as you can. Even if you are making pickles or salads, try to use as little salt as possible.

- **Shop for fresh veggies:** Avoid using canned and salted vegetables; instead, opt for fresh or frozen vegetables. Canned foods can be misleading because you might choose a tuna sandwich, thinking fish is a healthy option, but the brine and sauce that the tuna is packed in can make it heavy on calories and extremely high in sodium. The more you consume fresh meats, fruits, and vegetables, the healthier eating habits you will cultivate.

- **Wipe it off:** You can try a trick like "unsalting" your snacks. If you have a packet of salted and spiced nuts or seeds, you can always use a napkin to clean off the extra salt. Though we know it is best to not consume excessively salty foods, simple methods like this can come in handy when there are no other options. In fact, snacks are the most common means by which unregulated sodium enters your system. Imagine you are at work and your colleague offers you some salted nuts. Your first response might be to take them and munch on them, but it is very important to be wary of what you consume, regardless of the portion. Try keeping a stash of unsalted nuts at your desk!

- **Wash your food first:** Prior to cooking, make sure to rinse foods, including fruits, vegetables, meat products, nuts, and everything that can be washed. This is great for hygiene, and at the same time, it cleans off any salt on the food products. For example, when you plan to prepare a simple chicken salad, make sure to rinse the chicken thoroughly before cooking. This process of draining the salt water out can be very helpful in reducing any extra sodium content. It may sound like one more pain-in-the-butt step, but the amount of harmful sodium content you save yourself from is worth the effort.

- **Opt for homemade:** Use homemade sauces and dressings for your food and salads. This way, you can reduce almost half the sodium that would be present in prepackaged sauces and dressings. Often, when we dine out and order a vegetable salad, we assume that we are eating very healthy and nothing can go wrong but somehow end up bloated the next day. This happens because most of the salads prepared at restaurants are seasoned with sauces and vinegar that are loaded with sodium and various tastemakers. For example, the fish sauce that is used widely contains a whopping quantity of sodium!

- **Avoid artificial flavors:** Bottled and flavoring packets, like ready-made broth cubes, often contain monosodium glutamate (MSG). This is one of the main reasons why you often feel instantly thirsty after having food with a high sodium content, including MSG. Stick to using fewer artificial flavors to enhance the taste of your food. Always go for natural flavors, like garlic, spices, pepper, citrus juice, and salt-free condiments, while preparing food.

While reducing the sodium content in your food can be a great way to achieve your health goals, consuming healthy and natural foods can be much easier and is also one of the best ways to avoid unnecessary sodium. You might be doing all the relevant crunches and cardio to lose weight, but your tummy simply doesn't show any sign of improvement. Make sure to check how much sodium you have been consuming. You may be surprised to find that the quantity is much more than you think!

The bottom line is that no amount of heavy workouts will give you results if you are not watching your diet and salt intake. Eating organic and non-processed food, coupled with a few hours of physical activity a week, can do wonders for your waistline. Eating more fruits and vegetables can help you achieve a balance in your system and make you feel and look fitter in the long run, too.

A clean, well-rounded diet is not only good for your body but can also do wonders for your mind—another reason why checking what and how much is on your plate before you take that first bite is extremely important. Balanced food choices and proper quantities can make a big difference when multiplied day over day, week over week, and month over month. It all adds up, and consistency is key.

Some Salty Scoop!

Let's be honest, when we think of losing extra inches from our bellies, the first thing that comes to mind is cutting down on calories. But do we ever think about cutting out the salt completely? Not really! But there are a few top models in the glam world who swear by avoiding salt before their photoshoots. As a medical professional, I was flabbergasted by the thought of removing salt completely from the diet, as there could be many harmful health repercussions.

I further delved into this subject and discovered that many models follow something called a "salt depletion diet" a few days before their fashion shoots. I understand that sodium has a huge role in making you look and feel bloated and uncomfortable—along with the many other health issues it can cause, which we've already explored—but the dangers of abstaining from it completely are also a thing.

David Gandy, a male model, shared some of his secrets of preparing for a high-profile photoshoot for Dolce &

Gabbana. He mentioned that he adopted the salt depletion diet because salt caused bloating. Two days before a shoot, he would cut out salt from his diet, and then the day before the shoot, he would dehydrate himself by drinking only one glass of water the whole day and taking a hot water bath at night (NewBeauty Editors, 2017)! The whole point here was to have no water retention issue at the time of the shoot. I am giving this example because I, as a professional, intend to make everyone aware of how dangerous adopting such a diet plan can be. I find it so interesting what some professions/people will go through to achieve (completely unrealistic for the day-to-day gal) beauty standards.

However, I should highlight that while there are potential long-term negative effects of a fully "no salt" diet, this does not contradict the prior discussions in this chapter about limiting excessive salt intake. It is important to realize that neither too little nor too much salt is beneficial to your health. Anything done beyond a limit is dangerous.

Time and again, we are reminded of conventional beauty standards by fashion magazines and videos, which often make us doubt our fitness and appearance. That's another reason why prioritizing your health and mental peace is so, so important. Whether it is for your job or to "impress" someone, no amount of validation is worth your physical and mental health. It is the lifestyle that you choose and the healthy options of food and drink that you incorporate into your life that will help you gain a better perspective on health and fitness. Look better *and* feel better with moderate, healthful consistency.

Being aware of what you consume and in what quantity, understanding the role of sodium in your diet and weight issues, and adopting ways to stay fit and healthy is the best gift you can give yourself. When your mind and body start working in sync, you will notice that you start feeling fitter and fabulous in no time! Don't eliminate salt altogether; instead, use it sparingly and in accordance with your health. To become the best version of yourself and to work toward your flat belly, drink enough water, eat a balanced diet, move your body, and think optimistically.

Chapter 2:

Embracing Healthy Fats

The word "fat" has been made into something scary, hasn't it? Perhaps this is due to the widespread negative image of "fat" that has been propagated for a long time. The problem is the generalization of fats as something harmful, which creates a conflicting attitude toward the consumption of fats and their importance and risk in our diets.

I'm sure we all have been told to stay away from fat by our friends, family, colleagues, and the good old interwebs at times. If we learned anything from the 90s, it is that being on a "low fat" diet caused most of us to have weight problems for the first time. The "low fat" foods often substitute additional ingredients to boost flavor and taste that are far worse for us than if we had just left the naturally occurring fat *in*.

Healthy fats, such as polyunsaturated fats and monounsaturated fats, are required for a flat belly and many body operations. Consequently, a sufficient amount of fats should be included in your normal dietary intake for additional nutrition and its benefits. When we talk about fats, many patients are confused about how fats may be helpful and what various examples of fats exist in both of these categories of fat. Yes, it's understandable that distinguishing between healthy and "bad" fats might be tricky if you don't have the right information, so here you go!

Differentiating Between Good and Bad Fats

Fats can be difficult to understand, and for that reason alone, it is very important to have a clear picture of the differentiating factors between good and bad fats. Your health depends on the type of food you consume regularly, and making healthy food choices and habits can help you keep many diseases, especially cardiovascular disease, at bay.

When it comes to fat—or any type of food—overconsumption can be risky. However, eating the right food can be one of the best things you can do for your health and self-care. Let's learn what good fats and bad fats are so you can easily make healthy choices now and in the future.

How Did Fats Earn a Bad Reputation?

In the homes of older generations, having fat-laden food has been a topic of conversation for a long time. Plates full of bacon and eggs were easier to prepare and delicious to eat at the start of a busy and active day. Due to the high-calorie content, fats were traditionally regarded as one of the best sources of energy. The idea then was to consume tasty fats and stay full longer. It wasn't until researchers conducted several studies that we got the idea that some fats might be "good" and some might be "bad."

In the 1930s, Russian scientist Nikolai Anitchkov found that consumption of high cholesterol by animals could lead to a condition called atherosclerosis. In this condition, plaque accumulates in the arteries, constricting them and elevating the risk of heart disease, increasing the chances of heart attack (University of Minnesota, 2006).

Later, during the 1940s and 1950s, cases of cardiovascular disease decreased, which was credited to the wartime rationing system. So, the widespread notion that rich, high-fat food could be dangerous for the heart became common. Interestingly, researchers examined a group of men with similar characteristics and health conditions by monitoring their blood pressure, serum cholesterol, smoking habits, diet, alcohol consumption, and age. They observed that in about 15 years, deaths among these men were mostly from cardiovascular disease, followed by stroke and cancer. They saw that diverse risk factors, like obesity, high blood cholesterol, and hypertension, could be responsible for heart disease. Additionally, saturated fat in the diet was shown to increase cholesterol and, therefore, increase the risk of heart ailments (Keys et al., 1986).

The bottom line of this study was that not all types of fat posed risks, and not all fats were the same. However, over time, the concept and analysis were likely misrepresented, and the fear of any form of fat quickly spread worldwide. Because of widespread misinformation, it is crucial to dispel any misconceptions, get accurate information about everything you ingest, and understand the distinction between good and bad fats.

Good Fats

There are a whole bunch of fats that are great and do not pose any threat to your heart or overall health. These fats are so good for your health that they can even protect you from several ailments and also help lower your blood cholesterol levels.

Let's talk about the fats that are highly beneficial for your wellness. But note that eating too much of anything may be harmful, and because healthy fats also have a considerable amount of calories and triglycerides, consume them in moderation for the optimal outcome.

Here are some of the "good" fats you should include in your diet:

Unsaturated Fats

Unsaturated fats are healthy fats that are considered to be beneficial for your health. Saturated fats stay solid at room temperature, and unsaturated fats, like oil, stay liquid at the same temperature. This is one of the simplest methods to tell them apart. To avoid any confusion, it is also crucial to note that "trans fat" and "saturated fat" are bad types of fat for your body.

Here are a few of the benefits of unsaturated fats:

- They help provide fuel for the body.

- They help protect the organs of the body.

- They improve the absorption of nutrients in the system.

- They support the healthy growth of cells.

- They help produce vital hormones.

- They boost the level of high-density lipoprotein (HDL), which is also known as "good cholesterol."

- They help lower the risk of cardiovascular diseases.

Two of the most important types of unsaturated fats are monounsaturated and polyunsaturated fats.

Monounsaturated Fats

Monounsaturated fats (monounsaturated fatty acids, or MUFAs) stay liquid at room temperature but can turn semi-solid when kept in a very cold setting. Plant-based oils, like olive oil, canola oil, safflower oil, sesame oil, and canola oil, are some of the types of monounsaturated fats. Seeds, nuts, avocados, and peanut butter are also rich sources of this fat.

This type of fat can not only be helpful for your cells and heart but can also be beneficial for weight loss.

According to one study, when 124 obese people were given either a diet high in monounsaturated fats or a diet high in carbs for a year, on average, those who consumed monounsaturated fats lost more weight (Brehm et al., 2008).

Polyunsaturated Fats

Vegetable oils, like soybean, corn, cottonseed, sunflower, and safflower, are a few examples of polyunsaturated fats (polyunsaturated fatty acids, or PUFAs). Margarines, salad dressings, and mayonnaise also contain some of these fats. Polyunsaturated fats are liquid at room temperature and stay liquid even when refrigerated. Two of the most important types of polyunsaturated fats are omega-3 and omega-6 fatty acids. Consuming these fats and replacing saturated fats with them can help lower levels of bad cholesterol and boost levels of good cholesterol.

Among the two, omega-3 fatty acids are considered the best for health.

Omega-3 Fatty Acids

Omega-3s are polyunsaturated fats that are crucial for the body to function. These can be obtained only from diet and other supplements because the body is unable to produce them. They are an important part of the cell membranes, help provide structure and support, and further boost interaction among the cells.

A diet rich in omega-3 fatty acids reduces the risk of heart disease, blood clots, arrhythmia (abnormal heart rhythm), some types of cancer, dementia, Alzheimer's disease, and age-related macular degeneration. It also helps lower the triglyceride and cholesterol levels in the blood. Marine sources—fatty fish like salmon, mackerel, tuna, halibut, sardines, herring, pompano, sea bass, and lake trout—are rich in omega-3s. Also, walnuts, flaxseed, canola oil, soy products, and soybeans contain omega-3s to some extent (Cleveland Clinic, 2019).

Bad Fats

The fats that fall in the "bad" category are the ones you need to watch out for, including saturated fats. Saturated fats are solid at room temperature and are very high in low-density lipoprotein cholesterol (LDL), or bad cholesterol. These fats are also called "solid fats" and are some of the most common fats found in the American diet.

Saturated fats are found largely in animal fats and dairy products. Consumption of excessive saturated fat can increase bad cholesterol levels and raise the risk of high insulin resistance and heart diseases. Beef, poultry, pork, eggs, tropical oils (like palm and coconut), high-fat dairy products, and butter are some of the most common sources of saturated fats.

According to the World Health Organization's guidelines, it is essential to keep track of your fat intake to maintain good health. It is also important to follow the right "macro" count for your body. This is the ratio of carbohydrates, fat, and protein you consume daily.

You can find generic amounts online, or we can run a custom calculator for you based on your DNA when you visit www.lifelongmetaboliccenter.com.

Artificial trans fats in processed food were banned by the Food and Drug Administration in 2020 (Wellness & Prevention, 2023). Trans-fatty acids and saturated fats can be replaced by polyunsaturated and monounsaturated fats derived from plant sources. Intake of high artificial trans fats and saturated fats increases the risk of type 2 diabetes and heart disease.

How Healthy Fats Support a Flat Belly

When it comes to losing weight and dropping a few inches, people often turn to reducing their fat intake. As previously said, fat is not the sole enemy. While the bad form can lead to major issues, it may be difficult to believe, but good dietary fats can help you lose weight and get rid of stubborn belly fat!

Monounsaturated fats and omega-3 fatty acids are the real deal and can not only help you stay healthy but can also boost your fat loss journey at the same time. According to a study, the consumption of polyunsaturated fatty acids (PUFAs) raises your resting metabolic rate, which is the calorie consumption needed to live. Additionally, it also increases diet-induced calorie burn, which means that there is a higher and faster rate of calorie breakdown of PUFAs in comparison to saturated fats (News, 2012).

Here are a few interesting ways good fats can help achieve a flat belly (Palinski-Wade, 2016):

Extended Digestion

One of the most common reasons for weight gain is the consumption of more calories than needed for the body to function. Constant snacking due to hunger cravings can lead to a high appetite and result in overeating. Studies show how fats and satiety are related. For instance, healthy and balanced consumption of good fats can affect satiety and can even help in controlling appetite by releasing appetite hormones (Samra, 2010).

Research conducted by UC Irvine pharmacologists found that fatty foods like nuts, olive oil, and avocados help curb hunger by transmitting signals to the brain to prevent excessive eating. This theory is opening new doors in treating obesity and related eating disorders (Irvine, 2008).

Reduces Inflammation

Weight gain is often linked with elevated inflammation in the body, and vice versa. Inflammation is the body's natural defensive system, and prolonged inflammation is associated with serious medical conditions, including obesity. With high levels of inflammation, glucose concentration in the body increases, resulting in excessive fat formation as carbohydrates become harder to digest. As the metabolism slows down, the body's weight tends to creep up. As a result, losing extra pounds can be particularly challenging.

A controlled diet and, more so, an anti-inflammatory diet and a healthy lifestyle are needed to reduce inflammation. A well-balanced diet rich in proteins, fiber, and healthy fats such as olive oil, seafood, nuts, and seeds is advantageous. You can reduce the risk of heart disease and type 2 diabetes by avoiding bad fats, reducing alcohol use, and eating good fats regularly. Additionally, you can efficiently decrease belly fat as your energy increases and metabolism improves with an improved diet and effective lifestyle changes (Drop Bio Health, n.d.).

Reduces Stress Hormones

Prolonged stress and exhaustion could be the reasons behind the production of the stress hormone cortisol in the body. This is a common reason for an increase in fat around the belly and overall weight gain. Good fats, especially omega-3s, can help reduce stress hormones and help cut down extra fat from the body, mainly the belly region, at the same time (Palinski-Wade, 2016).

Incorporating Healthy Fats Into Your Diet

At this point, you are aware of precisely how important it is to include healthy fats in your diet every day to keep both your body and mind in good health. A variety of medical conditions, including those with signs and symptoms that have no known etiology, may have nutrition and food imbalance as their underlying cause. These include a persistent sense of exhaustion or lack of energy; dry skin, hair, and nails; shifts in mood; and, more often than not, weight gain or loss due to prolonged stress and anxiety.

A little planning and discipline are all you need to start a healthy lifestyle. Including good fats in your diet is not that big of a challenge, as most of the food products in that category taste quite good. Nuts, seeds, fatty fish, full-fat yogurt, cheese, and avocados are some splendid choices you can make to include good fats in your diet.

Here are a few ways you can incorporate healthy fats into your regular diet to reap maximum benefits:

- **Check the labels**: Always check the labels of food products to monitor how much fat is in the food you eat. You will be able to consume fat and monitor the quantity with this method.

- **Savor as you eat:** Eat food slowly and make sure to chew thoroughly. This will help in the breakdown of calories and also reduce your appetite by making you feel full, preventing overeating.

- **Monitor your portions:** It's important to control your portions while eating. For example, no matter how hungry you may be, try eating a healthy portion rather than stuffing yourself with excess food. Use a smaller plate to avoid grabbing too large of portions.

- **Stock up on healthy snacks:** Keep some nuts and seeds handy at home or work to snack on whenever you get hungry. This will prevent you from eating something unhealthy when hungry. You can purchase individual serving sizes to prevent overeating larger quantities without realizing it.

Fats are a great source of energy, and when you incorporate healthy fats into your diet, you will start noticing the difference in your health. They not only replenish your body and mind but are also helpful for your weight-loss journey. Knowing and counting your macros can be the best way to reduce belly fat and the heavy feeling in your body. Balance those good fats with an appropriate amount of carbohydrates and protein as well to get the most bang for your buck.

Cooking Techniques for Maximizing Benefits

If you have been wondering how to incorporate healthy fats into your home cooking, here are a few simple ways to create yummy food with great health benefits:

- **Garnish your food with seeds and nuts:** This can be an amazing way to increase nutrients and healthy fats. Sprinkle nuts or seeds over your favorite bowl of oatmeal in the morning or salad during the day. This will not only add a zing and flavor to your food but also benefit your overall health.

- **Use olive oil:** Olive oil is anti-inflammatory and considered to be extremely healthy. Every time you cook, drizzle some olive oil on it. Whether you are cooking sautéed vegetables, preparing pasta, or making some salad dressing, make sure to use olive oil for great health benefits.

- **Try canned fish:** Canned fish is an option for those with busy schedules who are also not very keen on cooking their meals. You can stock your fridge with canned seafood, like tuna and salmon, and use it while preparing food of your choice. Add some tuna to your sandwich and you will get a healthy dose of good fats along with a protein source. Trader Joe's carries canned tuna with zero added sodium.

- **Stock up on avocados:** Avocados are a great source of healthy fats and have many health benefits. Use fresh avocados to make toast, guacamole, or any food item of your choice. If available, try to include avocados in your diet regularly (Ball, 2022).

Planning Ahead

Preplanning is one of the most effective ways to stay on track with your goals. Incorporating healthy fats into your diet is similar, so one of the best methods to manage how much of each kind of food you consume is to prepare and organize your meals ahead of time. If you have your meals prepared, you'll not only take less time to decide what to eat, but you'll also be more mindful of what you put in your mouth.

You can precisely track your calorie intake in this manner, which will be very beneficial for your fitness and weight-loss goals. This is also great for those with busy lifestyles. Preplan according to your macros on Sunday. Shop, chop, and prep foods. Then, Monday through

Friday, just eat what you have planned. No thinking is needed during the busy work week!

Watch Your Weight With Fats

It's interesting to think about how fat might help you lose weight and shrink your waistline. In this chapter, I have drawn a clear picture of how there are distinct and different types of fats and that each has its role to play in either harming your health or protecting you from many conditions. How you want to feel can depend on what type of fat you choose to consume!

Fats act as a fuel that helps keep your body going, similar to carbohydrates and proteins. The famous Halle Berry, the 57-year-old actress, has many times shared her experience with trying a high-fat diet to stay fit and prevent diabetes. She is particular about having healthy fats, like avocados, on her plate daily. Similarly, LeBron James, the famous basketball star, also followed a high-fat diet to get his abs more ripped and healthy (Lawler, 2018).

Every person is unique in terms of their health conditions, food sensitivities, and metabolism levels, so it is extremely important to get the right plan for you.

Simple Exercises to Help Burn That Hard-To-Lose Belly Fat

The benefits of a healthy diet with the right amount of good fats are immense. However, when you add a few effective exercises to your routine, your journey from a flab belly to a flat belly can become much easier.

Here are a few workouts that can be super effective in the process:

Cardio or Aerobics

Belly fat, which is visceral fat, is more stubborn than fat in other areas. Doing cardio or aerobic exercise most days can help control your belly fat. Cardio exercises, like running, walking, rowing, swimming, cycling, and jogging, are known to burn a lot of calories, resulting in effective weight loss. However, if you have any underlying health issues, do not pressure yourself into trying difficult exercises.

Make sure to start slow and gradually increase the pace as much as your body can do safely. For those with health conditions, one of the best cardio exercises that never fails is simply walking! So, put those headphones on and take a brisk walk out in the park for a few minutes every single day. Enjoy the warm sunshine and fresh air and take some deep, cleansing breaths.

Weight Training

Weight training is highly beneficial for reducing belly fat. When combined with resistance training, these workouts can boost your metabolism and reduce your body fat. Squats, lunges, tricep kickbacks, and bicep curls are some exercises that show results effectively.

However, make sure to weight train using lighter weights at first, and only then gradually try heavier weights. Lifting weights can improve your metabolism, improve body composition, and burn more calories.

Abdominal Exercises

Like all the other exercises, you should start ab exercises gradually and then increase the intensity. Abdominal crunches, bicycle crunches, planks, and leg lifts are some of the most effective abdominal exercises.

Along with these, the practice of lower abdominal workouts can also be beneficial to boost your strength, posture, balance, and self-confidence. There are a few specific exercises, like mountain climbers, leg raises, scissor kicks, toe touches, and knee tucks, that have also proven to be highly effective in reducing belly fat.

Interval Training and High-Intensity Interval Training (HIIT)

High-intensity interval training, or HIIT, is a combination of intense and varied exercises. For example, during a workout, a very intense and difficult exercise is done for some time and then followed by something light and easy. Rest breaks are taken in between as well. For example, when you do HIIT, you will work on high-intensity movements for half a minute and then rest for another half a minute. This form of exercise is said to be very helpful in reducing belly fat and regulating your overall body weight.

Pulling, pushing, deadlifting, and squatting are some of the exercises that can fall under this category or the weightlifting category. If you do these intensely followed by breaks, they can help you lose a lot of weight. Similarly, exercises like jumping jacks, burpees, high knees, jump squats, and pushups are said to be equally effective in losing belly fat. When you do steady-state cardiovascular exercises, you burn more calories while you are doing the exercise. When you do a HIIT workout, you burn more calories than in the other 23 hours of the day.

Exercising provides innumerable health benefits. From preventing various diseases to increasing your energy, a good workout can give you peace of mind. An added bonus here is the weight and fat loss from the belly. It is natural that when you lose weight, it is quite difficult to lose weight only from a particular section. No, your calorie burners do not work that way and are not selective in cutting off the fat from your body only from the areas that you like (WebMD Contributors, 2023).

By performing "spot exercises" to the core and abdominal region, you give yourself the best chance at affecting that area. If you can fill it with muscle, it looks more tight and toned overall. The combo of proper macros and specific exercises is the best thing you can do for a fast flat belly.

Moreover, to lose weight, you do not have to have access to a fitness club. You can start working on your body right at home. Neither expensive equipment nor expensive diet foods are needed. Stay cautious and watch out for the red flags in the food that you consume. Lots of things that are available in the market are contaminated with artificial add-ons, so finding the right food and place to exercise every day is your best bet.

Eating the simplest of food and from the original sources is very helpful. For example, instead of opting for supplements for fats, nutrients, and vitamins, try to find the simplest and the easiest available natural food. We should eat the way your grandparents did—with maybe a bit less bacon (wink).

So, whether you plan to win a marathon or simply go for a walk in a quiet park, your fitness and holistic health play a major part in making your vision a reality. The bigger your belly gets, the higher your risk of developing unpleasant health conditions in the long run. No age is too late to start with a fitness goal, and regardless of where you are in life, physically or mentally, make sure to realize that it is *you* who you have to take good care of!

Start giving yourself the importance and love you have been giving others all your life. Work on your health goals now, and no matter your age, make sure to move on with a positive outlook. As you progress with this book, you will feel much more sorted and healthy, and in no time, you will be able to work on your mind and body in full swing. Prioritize yourself and embrace all the good things in life, starting with the "good" fats in your diet!

Chapter 3:

Managing Gaseous Foods

We live in a progressive era that, to a great extent, is committed to diversity, inclusiveness, and optimism. Across the globe, there are different types of people with varied skin colors, cultures, body types, health conditions, and even mindsets. Everyone's bodies are not the same, neither are the ways their bodies react to different types of foods and environments. However, one thing that is quite common worldwide is the problem of gaseous foods and the related issues with bloating, which can contribute to severe discomfort.

We all have moments when we do not feel our best, even if we work out regularly and eat clean. There will be days when you wake up feeling bloated, and just when you plan to wear your favorite outfit, it may suddenly feel a tad tight and uncomfortable. Yes, bloating is real and can be extremely problematic at times. We can't deny that there are certain foods and food products that we may be consuming without even realizing that they could be the reason behind those recurring gaseous moments and bloated days!

What Is Gas and Bloating?

Gas and bloating are parts of the very normal process of digestion. Trapped gas can be extremely painful and is also known as gas pain. Though bloating may not be painful, it does generate a feeling of snugness and unease. The feeling of being puffed up, which can be visible as well, can give a blow to your mental and physical state. Burping, belching, and passing gas are some of the most natural processes that help release unnecessary gas from the body.

Digestive issues can be caused by many underlying health conditions. Aerophagia, the excessive swallowing of air, is one condition, but the food you consume can be one of the biggest culprits. That's why it's vital to gain correct information and create a clear understanding of the foods that can cause such issues. By doing so, you can work on reducing the symptoms and find ways to gain permanent relief from the pain and discomfort caused by digestive issues.

Identifying Common Gas-Inducing Foods

One of the first steps to help control gas formation in your stomach is to keep track of what you eat, when you eat, and how much you eat. Once again, food journaling comes into play. Many types of food are gas-inducing.

Your susceptibility to gas and bloating depends on your tolerance level for these foods. If you have been suffering from gas and problems related to it for some time, here are a few things to watch out for:

Cruciferous Vegetables

Vegetables must, without a doubt, be a regular part of a well-rounded diet. There may be times when you're maintaining a healthy diet and limiting your intake of unhealthy items, but despite your efforts, you still experience flatulence troubles. This might imply that you need to keep track of the vegetables you routinely eat. Many vegetables, such as cruciferous vegetables, have a reputation for causing abdominal discomfort and gas.

Brussels sprouts, cabbage, broccoli, cauliflower, asparagus, bok choy, radishes, watercress, arugula, collard greens, and the like are cruciferous vegetables. When consumed, these high-fiber vegetables can be difficult to digest, which is likely to cause gas formation. These vegetables have oligosaccharides, a form of sugar, called raffinose, which is not present in the human system, making it difficult to break down. Some cruciferous vegetables get digested when they enter the small intestine, but when they enter the large intestine, they do not get digested, causing gas to develop.

Additionally, glucosinolates, or chemicals containing sulfur that are found in these vegetables when broken down in the intestine, form hydrogen sulfide and cause a pungent smell like sulfur when gas is passed (Cording, 2018). Though cruciferous vegetables are rich in nutrients and vitamins, we can't overlook the fact that they play a significant part in causing gas and bloating.

Legumes and Beans

Ever wonder why devouring a meal that includes beans and legumes makes your stomach bloated? Well, the beans and legumes are to blame, not you, if you experience just the slightest bit of farting after eating! Fermentable fibers called oligosaccharides are found in beans, similar to those of cruciferous vegetables, which are hard to digest and can cause gas and bloating.

Fiber can cause bloating, flatulence, and stomach pain. Although a high-fiber diet has numerous health advantages, it can also have some negative effects if it is abruptly consumed in large amounts. For example, if you decide to include a large bowl of a certain bean in your diet all of a sudden, then your body will react, causing gas and bloating because it will take time to get used to it. However, if you consume beans frequently, your body may become acclimated to them, and your gas problems may eventually disappear (Cleveland Clinic, 2023).

Studies show that certain beans, like black-eyed peas, pinto beans, and vegetarian baked beans, can cause more flatulence than other beans. Lentils, broad beans, chickpeas, and peas are some of the other food items that cause bloating. The prime reason behind this could be that people have varying tolerance levels for different beans (Winham & Hutchins, 2011).

Bloating and gas issues can be highly uncomfortable and can affect your everyday life. Apart from fiber-rich items, like legumes and beans, some dairy products, whole-grain cereals, some fruits and vegetables, and even chewing gum can add to the problem of indigestion and gas formation. However, it's not advisable to avoid fiber-rich and nutrient-rich foods like these because of their many other health benefits. It is best to go ahead and eat these good-for-you foods, but find a solution to reduce the bloating and gas.

Here are a few ways you can do so:

- **Walk:** Walking can improve blood circulation and bowel movements, making it very effective at reducing gas. Try taking a walk after every meal to reduce flatulence and digestive issues.

- **Practice yoga:** There are numerous yoga poses that can help release gas from the gastrointestinal tract. Child's pose, squats, and happy baby pose can all be very beneficial for releasing gas and minimizing bloating.

- **Try an over-the-counter solution:** Anti-gas pills and medications are available to reduce gas and its effects. Peppermint capsules are also commonly used to relieve gas and bloating. However, medication should be taken only with a medical practitioner's consultation.

- **Utilize essential oils:** The use of certain essential oils, like curcumin and fennel, is effective in reducing bloating and gas. Use them in proportions that are recommended by a professional to avoid any side effects.

- **Relax:** Gentle massage on the abdomen, a warm bath, and other relaxation methods can be very helpful in reducing the symptoms of gas and bloating.

- **Use digestive enzymes:** Having a digestive enzyme like Beano with these foods can help your body digest them with less or even sometimes no gaseous effect.

Additionally, adopting a healthy lifestyle, eating healthy food, and staying hydrated at all times can help reduce bloating problems. For example, taking probiotics, reducing sodium intake, and avoiding only those gas-prone food items for *you* can be great for your overall well-being. Lifelong Metabolic Center offers a fab probiotic if you are interested in beginning to take one on a regular basis.

Although the vast majority might not perceive gas and bloating problems as serious, it's crucial to understand when you should see a medical professional.

Here are a few symptoms that you should watch out for:

- diarrhea

- fever

- vomiting

- appetite loss or gain

- abdominal pain

- weight loss

- blood in stool

Bloating can also be caused by water retention problems that could subside with adequate water intake in a few days. However, if the above symptoms continue for an extended time, then you need to visit your doctor as soon as possible.

Understanding Digestive Processes

The human digestive system consists of the gastrointestinal tract (GI tract), also called the digestive tract, and organs, such as the gallbladder, pancreas, and liver. The digestive tract is also made up of hollow organs comprising the mouth, esophagus, stomach, small intestine, large intestine, and anus.

All of these organs function together to break down the consumed food into nutrients and energy. These nutrients enter the bloodstream and help the cells in the body repair and grow. The food is broken down into different parts, such as carbohydrates, fats, vitamins, and proteins, which have specific functions in the body.

Digestion is highly crucial for the body to operate and stay healthy. For example, it is through the digestive process that proteins are broken down into amino acids, carbohydrates into sugar, and fats into glycerol and fatty acids. So, how does the digestive process work? Let's dive into a few specifics to understand it clearly:

When you consume food, your actions and motions, like chewing, mixing, and squeezing, help break down the food. The digestive juices, enzymes, stomach acid, and bile play a major role in digestion.

Here are examples of how each organ in the digestive system helps in the digestion process:

- **Mouth:** The digestive tract starts with the mouth. The saliva, which is a digestive juice, helps soften the food that you eat and also helps break down the food.

- **Esophagus:** Once the food is chewed in the mouth, the peristalsis helps push the food farther down through the esophagus and into the stomach.

- **Stomach:** The stomach lining has glands that produce enzymes and stomach acid, which play a huge role in breaking down food.

- **Pancreas:** The pancreas produces the enzymes that are responsible for the breakdown of proteins, fats, and carbohydrates. Additionally, it helps deliver the digestive juices to the small intestine through ducts, which are small tubes.

- **Liver:** The liver produces bile and pancreatic juice, which helps in digesting lipids and vitamins. Bile is transported through bile ducts from the liver to the gallbladder and the small intestine.

- **Gallbladder:** The gallbladder helps store bile in between food consumption. It also helps squeeze bile through the bile ducts to the stomach while food is being eaten.

- **Small intestine:** The small intestine produces digestive juices that amalgamate with pancreatic juice and bile and helps in the digestion of proteins, fats, and carbohydrates. The microbiome, or the bacteria in the intestine, also further helps in the digestion of carbohydrates.

- **Large intestine:** The bacteria in the large intestine helps digest nutrients and also helps make vitamin K.

- **Anus:** After digestion is completed, waste products become stool and are secreted through the anus, completing the entire digestive process.

The nutrients in the body are mostly absorbed by the small intestine. The circulatory system of the body transfers nutrients to various other parts of the system. Glucose, fatty acids, amino acids, and glycerol are some of the substances that are needed by the body to grow, repair the cells, and get energy (*Your Digestive System & How It Works*, 2023).

How Gas Is Produced in the Digestive Tract

Because there are multiple possible causes of gas formation in the digestive tract, let's explore it in more detail (*Symptoms & Causes of Gas in the Digestive Tract*, n.d.):

- **Swallowed air:** As we already know, when you swallow more air than normal, it can cause gas and gas symptoms. This can be caused by chewing gum, drinking carbonated drinks, eating quickly, smoking, and even wearing loose-fitted dentures.

- **Bacteria in the intestine:** The gut microbiome in your system comprises countless bacteria, fungi, and viruses that play a significant role in digestion. The bacteria in the large intestine helps in the breakdown of carbohydrates. However, food items with high concentrations of starch, fiber, and sugar are difficult to digest, which causes gas formation.

- **Health conditions:** Many preexisting and underlying health conditions can be the reason why gas forms more frequently. Celiac disease, constipation, gastroparesis, gastroesophageal reflux disease, obstruction in the GI tract, lactose intolerance, dietary fructose intolerance, and ovarian, colorectal, or stomach cancer are some of the diseases that are said to cause gas problems.

Though gas problems are more common than we can imagine and not always caused by severe health problems, it is always a good idea to consult a doctor if symptoms like constipation, abdominal pain, weight loss, or diarrhea persist for a long period of time.

Strategies for Minimizing Gassiness

It is natural to crave foods that cause gas issues, but even the thought of their aftermath can be distressing. However, some of the so-called "gaseous" foods can be prepared in such a way that they do not produce gas when eaten. Though it may sound tedious, with a few tweaks to the food you prepare and other techniques, it is possible.

For example, in many households, legumes are soaked overnight before being cooked the next day. This is done not only to make the legumes softer but to also reduce the compounds in the food that can cause flatulence and indigestion. This is the case for some cruciferous vegetables, too. Cauliflower, for instance, is boiled or steamed, and the water is drained to further cook or just stir-fry it.

Numerous herbs and condiments are known to reduce bloating and gas. For example, probiotics and even herbs with carminative properties, like ginger, rosemary, fennel, sage, oregano, basil, clove, coriander, peppermint, and cumin, can be extremely beneficial in reducing gas issues. By incorporating these herbs and spices while cooking food, you can reduce flatulence and bloating. Similarly, chamomile, caraway, spearmint, parsley, and dill are considered great options for maintaining a healthy gut.

Apart from these natural remedies, sitting up straight during and after eating, taking a walk after a meal, eating frequent but smaller portions, drinking water at room temperature, and eating slowly are some easy ways to curb gas problems. Most of the medication for gas contains activated charcoal, simethicone, and galactosidase, which help in the digestion of food. Some people rely on these medications, and there are others who do not find them effective (Dallas, 2023).

Another interesting way to boost your digestive health is by combining foods! Our food consists mostly of proteins, carbohydrates, and fats. Proteins are digested somewhat slowly, carbohydrates are digested quickly, and fat is digested the slowest of all.

Here are a few points to note about combining foods for improved digestion (Troupe, 2018):

- **Don't mix starch and protein:** Try to avoid starches and protein together if possible. Though it is such a normal and tasty combination, eating a steak with loaded mashed potatoes can aggravate your flatulence problems.

- **Always include veggies:** Try to include vegetables even if you are cooking any form of protein, like meat, fish, cottage cheese, etc. This combination of foods is easy for digestion and lowers gas issues.

- **Eat fruit separately:** Mixing fruits in juice form together or with vegetables may not be a good idea. Consume fruit separately without mixing it with other meals. Ensure to eat melons separately.

- **Rely on good fats:** Healthy fats are great for your health and can be paired with numerous food items.

Observing and understanding your food is very important, and keeping a journal of what food triggered your gas can be beneficial in the long run, too. Avoiding it and calling it natural every time you puff some gas out of your body will not win friends and influence people.

Is Your Weight-Loss Diet Making You Gassy?

I intend to provide genuine information to everyone reading this and support you on your route to fitness using my expertise and experiences collected over the years. I'm sure there are several people who have been giving their heart and soul to reducing weight but are facing the typical hurdle of simply feeling gassy or rather sick every time they eat healthy food. You know that everything on that diet plate is healthy, yet there must be something that is just aggravating the situation and being of no help in the process.

To better grasp the situation, consider the following causes that could be making your diet problematic:

The "Diet" Foods

You enter the supermarket and hit the food section, and the most common site that you see these days is the endless number of aisles, all stocked up with low-calorie, no-fat, and all kinds of "diet foods." In the same context, the number of sugar-free and different sugar substitute options is way too many to confuse a hurried shopper like me! Well, a hidden culprit for your gas troubles could be found among those highly advertised and modified foods.

For example, if you are trying to reduce your sugar intake and opting for many of these sugar substitute items, then the gas you are experiencing may be because of your intolerance to sugar alcohols, which are also called polyols. They contain fewer calories than normal sugar and are used generously in sugar-free items, like bars and crackers, diet soda, and even yogurt. They can be found in numerous diet food items, and when you overconsume these items assuming they are healthy and not harmful, you often end up feeling sick.

These low-calorie sweeteners are not easily digested because they cause bloating, gas formation, and many other digestive issues, including diarrhea. There are a few fruits and vegetables that are said to contain sugar alcohols, and they, too, can cause gas and bloating. Some of the fruits and vegetables that contain natural sugar alcohols are apples, sweet potatoes, mushrooms, pears, and plums.

So, if you have been facing a challenge to lose weight because your weight issues are making you uncomfortable and sick most of the time, you can do the following:

- **Limit artificial sweeteners**: If you are used to having artificial sweeteners and sugar alcohols, then make an effort to eliminate your intake.

- **Look for hidden ingredients:** Check the labels of all the diet-friendly foods that you intend to consume, as there could be hidden calories, preservatives, and excessive sodium that could worsen your weight issues.

- **Avoid problem foods:** Check for all the items mentioned before in this section and avoid having those in your regular diet.

- **Rely on natural sweeteners:** Use natural sweeteners like honey or small amounts of good old-fashioned real sugar.

Always remember, anything eaten in moderation should be fine. So, instead of buying "diet foods," eat more home-cooked, naturally occurring food or organic options but with portion control (Plowe, 2022).

Fiber

This might sound out of place in this list, but it is a fact that too much fiber in your diet can become a bit difficult to digest. It is always advised to have fiber-rich food when on a weight-loss plan. It helps you stay satiated for a long period and is also nutritious. For example, kidney beans, when eaten in the morning, can make you feel full the rest of the day, which helps reduce your intake of unnecessary calories.

Fruits and vegetables, like pears, strawberries, blueberries, blackberries, oats, carrots, beets, broccoli, chia seeds, bananas, dark chocolates, and cruciferous vegetables, are some of the most common fiber-rich foods you can have while on a diet or to maintain a healthy lifestyle.

So, the dilemma remains: We know how healthy fiber-rich foods are and how often it is advised to have them while trying to lose weight, but how can they be causing extra weight gain and preventing you from reducing those belly inches?

Though the USDA advises including around 25 to 30 grams of fiber in your diet daily, many people often fail to consume the amount of fiber their bodies need. Most of us often run with a fiber-deficit condition without even realizing it. In this situation, when you enter a diet routine and start consciously adding more fiber to your diet, that can lead to more probable weight gain than weight loss.

No doubt, fiber is good for your health, but when consumed in the wrong way, it can create a few problems, like the one mentioned above. Refrain from adding fiber all of a sudden to your diet; rather, do it more gradually. Your body has to adjust to the way fiber-rich food gets added to your system. By understanding this concept of introducing fiber to your system, you will be able to make more effective diet plans and see the best results out of them (Plowe, 2022).

Carbonated Drinks and Juices

Carbonated drinks, like soft drinks, energy drinks, and juices, can be extremely tempting to quench your thirst. Time and again, the importance of drinking adequate water is laid out by experts and medical practitioners. From flushing out waste and toxins from the body and maintaining a normal body temperature to lubricating the joints and keeping you hydrated at all times, the benefits of water cannot be overstated.

Dietitians recommend drinking plenty of water while on a weight-loss plan. However, it has become more of a trend to juice and call it "healthy." It is better to have the full fruit than a blended version of it. Because of this, nutritionists often advise their patients and clients to refrain from drinking juice.

Though advised not to, one of the main reasons why people get tempted to drink carbonated drinks in place of water is because water can get bland and is tasteless. On the other hand, juice, soft drinks, and soda tend to quench your thirst and reduce cravings. If you are a fan of juicing, try to use the complete fruit. The skin of an apple plus the "guts" create a perfect blend of fiber/juice for great digestion and a slower "burn."

Every sip of a carbonated beverage taken through a straw doubles the likelihood of flatulence. This happens because the air bubbles in the drinks are taken in, allowing more air to enter the mouth and cause gas issues. The only way to reduce the ill effects of carbonated drinks is to refrain from them. Instead, you can opt for flavored water with fruits and herbs. Make sure to have unsweetened drinks because it is the hidden calories in foods and drinks that often go unnoticed and contribute to more weight gain and water retention problems.

Working out and controlling your diet will be much easier with a healthy body and mind. Once your bloating and gas formation is treated, it will be much easier for you to focus on losing weight, feeling more confident, and getting much healthier in the long term (Plowe, 2022).

More on Raffinose

Raffinose is an oligosaccharide, a tiny sugar molecule that is found in many vegetables, like Brussels sprouts, beans, broccoli, cabbage, and even whole grains. It is composed of complex carbohydrates, and it also has fructose, glucose, and galactose, all different sugar molecules. Since it is found in some of the most nutritious food sources, it cannot be said that it is bad; it is only when consumed more than needed that it can have side effects like upset stomach, digestion problems, and gas issues.

If you notice that some of the foods containing raffinose are impacting your weight-loss efforts and causing digestion issues as well, you can slow down the consumption of these foods. Instead of completely cutting off these food sources from your diet, you can gradually introduce them and slowly increase the quantity so your body does not react to a sudden change (Plowe, 2022).

Being aware of what you consume and in what portion can be beneficial in your weight-loss journey as well. More often than not, when you are on a journey of weight loss and reducing some weight off the abdomen, being sure of what you eat and what foods can create chaos in your system is very important. As we've seen, there are foods that fall into the category of gassy foods, which can make you feel heavier, bloated, and down. Identifying the foods that trigger your body and brain can help you sail toward achieving your fitness goals.

Regardless of whether you want to prevent or cure a certain illness or lose weight in general, making an effort to understand your body and its response to various types of food and situations is the best approach that you can take in your self-care journey. So, whether you want to lose some belly fat or stop those embarrassing flatulence episodes every now and then, paying attention to the food you consume regularly can be a life-changing experience altogether. By tracking these foods, you can keep in all of the healthy choices that work well with your body and reduce those that cause bloating for you—all working toward your flat belly.

Chapter 4:

Food Allergies and

Sensitivities

Doesn't everybody know that one kid who is allergic to *everything*?! You can't have PB and J at the lunch table because Adam might sit there next period. One food might be perfectly fine for one person and cause a horrific reaction in another. Therefore, it's necessary to recognize the difference between food sensitivities and allergies.

Recognizing Allergic Reactions and Sensitivities

When it comes to food allergies and food sensitivities, both conditions are the immune system's response to some of the foods we consume. Though both conditions appear to be similar, they can be completely different with regard to their symptoms.

Food Allergy

Allergic reactions to food include symptoms like itching, rashes, anaphylaxis, dizziness, swelling, and hives. Food allergies are caused by a response of the immune system and can be dangerous at times. Some of the most common foods that can cause allergies are eggs, soy, milk, shellfish, nuts, and wheat. The allergy can appear within a short period of time, and immediate medical help is required for severe symptoms.

For instance, I recall a day when all of my friends and I were enjoying a small picnic near the lake in the city. Music and laughter filled the air, but none of us imagined that the relatively simple dish we were eating could be so hazardous or that Raul, a friend of ours, would take a mouthful of it without knowing what was coming. It was a basic sauce with a few ground peanuts in it, and it turned out that Raul was allergic to peanuts. We were aware that he was allergic, but we had no idea that the sauce contained a peanut combination. Without wasting any time, we called for help and managed to take him to the emergency room on time! That was one of the scariest instances that I've come across to date.

Signs and Symptoms of Food Allergy

Serena Williams, the world-renowned American professional tennis star, and Brian Matusz, an American professional baseball pitcher, are both allergic to peanuts! Steve Martin, the famous American actor, writer, musician, and comedian, is allergic to shellfish, and Bill Clinton, the 42nd president of the United States, is said to be allergic to flour and chocolate! (Nohe, 2020). Food allergies can be clingy, quite difficult to get rid of without proper medication and care, and can happen to almost anyone. If not recognized and taken care of at the right time, they can lead to serious problems.

Countless people are allergic to one thing or another. However, serious food allergies can be lethal, so having a clear understanding of the allergens that affect you and the people around you can be of great help during emergencies.

Here are a few common signs and symptoms of a food allergy:

- having a tingling sensation and itching in the mouth

- sudden development of hives, rashes, and even eczema

- swelling of the lips, mouth, tongue, face, throat, and other parts of the body

- nasal congestion, breathing difficulty, wheezing conditions

- unexplained abdominal pain, nausea, diarrhea, and vomiting

- change in voice and difficulty swallowing food

- lightheadedness, dizziness, and even passing out or fainting

- a sudden drop in blood pressure, palpitation, and rapid pulse

The symptoms of a food allergy can vary; sometimes, they can last for just a few minutes, and at other times, they can last for a few hours. Symptoms like swelling of the tongue can be extremely dangerous, as it can cause obstruction and tighten the airways for breathing. In many cases, a few signs are so mild that people often do not realize that they are getting an allergic reaction. However, in some cases, the signs may be strong and can cause a person to weaken and lose consciousness in a matter of a few minutes (*Food Allergy*, 2021).

Visit a Doctor

If you notice even a slight allergic reaction, it is best to visit a doctor to understand the condition. Watch out for triggers every time you eat something that makes you feel uncomfortable. Most importantly, if you have signs, especially shortness of breath, constriction of airways, and rapid drop of blood pressure, then you must immediately rush to the nearest emergency room.

Diagnosis of Food Allergy

There are a few points the doctor will investigate when diagnosing a food allergy. In addition to going over your detailed medical history and your family's allergy history, here are a few questions they might ask:

- How long does it take for your allergy symptoms to develop?

- What food are you sensitive or allergic to?

- What are the primary signs that you experience when you have an allergic reaction?

These are some of the most common queries that almost every medical professional will make to understand your situation. However, as a responsible individual, you can keep track of which medications or foods you know you are allergic to and ensure that you provide accurate information to your doctor.

Tests for Food Allergies

Tests and examinations for food allergies are typically skin and blood tests. Medical professionals perform these tests to get a clear analysis of your specific allergies. Also, if you want to know what food is giving you allergies, then there are allergy testing methods that can help you understand your condition.

An allergist or medical professional will ask you various questions like the ones mentioned above about your allergies. This is one of the ways they will recognize what food items are giving you allergic reactions. However, simply performing an allergy test will not solve your problems. It takes dedication and effort on your end as well to prevent and work on your food allergy issues.

Here are the three most common tests that medical professionals conduct while figuring out food allergy conditions:

- **Skin test:** This is considered to be the quickest way to figure out food allergies. A drop of liquid is placed on the skin, and it is pricked with a needle. After waiting for some time, the doctor will observe any reaction, like the formation of a small bump or redness, to be sure of an allergic reaction. If the red bump resembles a mosquito bite, then that can indicate that you are allergic to the food. In the same test, if your skin does not react in any way, then that indicates you are not allergic to the food. This food allergy test can be performed on several food items.

- **Blood test:** It is a method used to find out about food allergies. A medical professional will take some blood and then be exposed to various allergens. The test sample is taken to the laboratory, and the result is awaited. Most doctors do not encourage this way of testing for allergies because it takes almost a week to get the reports back from the laboratories. However, it is said that tests like this and even the skin test are not completely foolproof and can have different results.

- **Controlled food challenge:** This is a test that is not used by doctors often. It is said to be harmful to people with chronic allergies. This is done in rare cases where the doctor gives a few samples and waits for any reaction to pinpoint the exact food that is causing the food allergies. It is because of this procedure that this method is considered to be unsafe and risky. However, you should opt for this option only when you are physically present in a medical facility where, even if something goes haywire, it can be controlled by experts (WebMD Editorial Contributors, 2022).

To find a solution to a problem, it is always a good idea to acknowledge the existence of a problem first. In the same way, your allergies can be handled and taken care of only when you recognize the main factor that is the root cause. Correct diagnosis and proper tests are of utmost importance.

Food Sensitivity

Food sensitivity, also called food intolerance, includes symptoms like gas, bloating, constipation, diarrhea, nausea, and cramps. Food intolerance is not caused by an immune response but by the body's inability to digest a certain type of food. Additionally, it is not a life-threatening condition. It is more like feeling gassy after having a bite of cheese or getting a severe toothache after having something sweet.

Food is a necessity, and staying away from various types of food can be impossible. There may be many times when we eat something for the first time without realizing we are sensitive to it. So, being cautious of what we eat and observing what foods cause sensitivity and allergy issues is vital. There are many tests that can check the causes of different allergies and sensitivities and treatments for them as well.

Effects of Untreated Allergies on Digestive Health

Allergies can be more than just painful; they can be highly irritating and also impact your regular life. From severe rashes and teary eyes to swollen faces or life-threatening reactions, one small negligence in what you eat can leave you bedridden for a long time. Consider a situation where you are allergic to pollen, but you can't avoid passing through the park or ignoring someone handing you a bouquet of flowers. You can imagine the scenario after that: messy, sickening, and frustrating! Well, in this case, the histamine causes this chaos. However, when it comes to food, it can be extra tricky to understand what is causing an allergic reaction, especially if you've never had one before.

Allergies can adversely affect the digestive system. Food allergies are linked to the gastrointestinal system because the first organ that the food you consume enters is the gastrointestinal tract. Many allergic reactions to the wrong food cause symptoms like abdominal pain, vomiting, and diarrhea. Also, when adopting a healthy lifestyle and losing weight, you often tend to try new types of dietary foods and supplements. Make note of any food that gives you even a slight sign of an allergy, especially when consuming it for the first time.

Studies show that more than 170 food items cause food allergies (*Food Allergy Versus Food Intolerance*, 2019). If undiagnosed and untreated, allergies can affect your digestive health, as around 70% of the immune system is present in the human gut (*Do Allergies Affect Your Gastro Health?* 2023). This makes it highly possible that the cause of your excessive bloating and gas formation could be allergies.

Inflammation and Digestive Discomfort

Inflammation in the gastrointestinal tract could be one of the biggest reasons for digestive discomfort and abdominal bloat. It is one of the primary aspects of the body's immune response. Depending on the duration, symptoms, and level of pain, inflammation can be called either chronic or acute inflammation. Irritable bowel disease (IBD), irritable bowel syndrome (IBS), gastroenteritis, gastroesophageal reflux disease (GERD), along with many other conditions that cause heat, pain, swelling, etc., are some of the inflammation that affects the digestive system.

No doubt, several health conditions are associated with inflammation in the digestive tract, causing discomfort and pain. Crohn's disease and ulcerative colitis are two of the most common health issues connected with IBD:

- Crohn's disease causes inflammation in the digestive tract, and it can affect the areas starting from the mouth to the anus. Pain in the abdomen, fever, loss of appetite, fatigue, weight loss, uneasy bowel movements, and watery and bloody diarrhea are some of its symptoms.

- Ulcerative colitis is an inflammatory bowel disease that begins in the rectum region and moves upward to the colon area. This condition is limited only to the rectum and colon. Diarrhea, discomfort, abdominal pain, and rectal bleeding are some of its symptoms.

Inflammation in any region can be a painful experience, and if the inflammation in the GI tract is not taken care of, then prolonged issues can even lead to the risk of bowel cancer.

Additionally, here are a few more conditions that can add to the problem of inflammation:

Irritable Bowel Syndrome (IBS)

Irritable bowel syndrome is a condition that affects the digestive tract, and many people get severe symptoms. It is a common issue and has to be taken care of medically. Symptoms of IBS are abdominal pain, cramps, bloating, diarrhea, gas, constipation, changes, and irregularity in bowel movement.

The primary causes of IBS are not limited to a single factor. It could be caused due to the following reasons:

- **Infection:** Excessive growth of bacteria can cause bouts of diarrhea and related infections in the intestines. This condition, called gastroenteritis, can be one of the main reasons for IBS problems.

- **Muscle contraction:** The muscles that line the intestine walls contract as the food passes through them. This is a normal digestive process, but if the contraction lasts longer and gets stronger, then various issues, like diarrhea, bloating, and gas, can be the result. On the contrary, if the contraction of the muscles gets slower than normal, then constipation and dry and hard stool can cause severe discomfort and problems.

- **Nerve issues:** The nervous system plays a significant role in the functioning of the digestive system by transmitting signals. However, when the transfer of signals weakens and the connection between the intestine and the brain gets disrupted or very slow, it can adversely affect the digestive process. Some of the symptoms caused by such factors are stomach aches, constipation, and even diarrhea.

- **Stress:** People with high stress levels from an early age are said to experience IBS symptoms more frequently.

- **Gut changes:** Changes in the gut microbiome with alterations in the level and type of bacteria, fungi, and viruses present in the intestine have an impact on the overall health of a person. It has been found that people with IBS have slightly different microbes than those without the condition.

It is vital to consult with your doctor if you experience excessive weight loss, night diarrhea, anemia or iron deficiency, rectal bleeding, or vomiting and if the pain does not subside even after taking over-the-counter medications. Depending on the severity of the condition, your doctor can give you medication or counseling treatments. The good news is that the risk of developing colorectal cancer and alteration in bowel tissue is minimal in this condition (*Irritable Bowel Syndrome*, n.d.).

Gastroesophageal Reflux Disease (GERD)

Gastroesophageal reflux disease is a condition caused by consistent stomach acid that moves back into the tube that connects your mouth and stomach. With GERD, there are moments when you eat something, and after a while, instead of getting a regular burp, you feel the acid from your stomach rise up through your digestive pipe and reach your mouth. This condition is often referred to as acid reflux and can be taxing to your esophagus.

Acid reflux is a normal and common condition most people experience. It can happen mostly after consuming rich, oily, and spicy food. However, if acid reflux gets too frequent, it becomes GERD, which can be controlled by simple lifestyle changes and medications.

Here are a few symptoms to watch out for:

- regurgitation or backwash of food or bitter liquid from the pipes of the intestine to the mouth

- uneasiness and a burning sensation like heartburn in the chest, mostly after eating something

- chest and upper abdominal pain

- dysphagia, the condition of difficulty swallowing

- a feeling of something stuck in the throat

Asthma disorders can also develop as a result of acid reflux at night, which can cause a persistent cough, laryngitis (pain/strain in the voice cords), and other respiratory problems. If any of these symptoms persist for a prolonged period, you should visit your doctor (*Gastroesophageal Reflux Disease (GERD)*, 2023).

Infectious Gastroenteritis

This condition is also referred to as the stomach flu. The inflammation in the stomach and the intestine is caused by bacteria, which further causes vomiting and diarrhea. Some of the most common symptoms of gastroenteritis are stomach aches, watery diarrhea, fever, nausea, cramping, and headache. This condition can also cause mild to severe dehydration, which can lead to lightheadedness, extreme thirst, and dry skin and mouth.

Gastroenteritis is infectious, as it can spread from someone suffering from the condition due to the virus, contaminated water and food, unhygienic conditions, changing diapers, unwashed hands, etc. Rotavirus and norovirus are the two most common types of the virus responsible for the condition. Though very rare, there are some parasites that can also cause gastroenteritis. Swimming in public pools and drinking contaminated water can be huge risk factors for parasites.

There are a few not very common but probable ways to get infectious gastroenteritis, like through the toxins present in certain seafood; excessive consumption of acidic foods; like tomatoes and citrus; metals present in drinking water; and various medications, like antibiotics, laxatives, antacids, and even chemotherapy drugs.

Drinking lots of fluids and gradually hydrating can be helpful. As symptoms like vomiting and diarrhea start subsiding, healthy eating is very important. Avoiding alcohol, dairy, and caffeine is important as well. However, if the symptoms persist and you face severe fatigue and weakness, you should consult with your doctor (DiLonardo, 2018).

Leaky Gut Syndrome (LGS)

Leaky gut syndrome is more of a hypothetical condition, and some doctors do not recognize LGS as a disease that is diagnosed. In this intestinal condition, bacteria, toxins, and food particles go past the intestinal lining into the bloodstream, which can lead to the weakening of the permeability of the intestinal walls, imbalance in the gut flora or microbiome, and further cause several diseases like Crohn's.

Some of the symptoms associated with this condition are constipation, acute diarrhea, bloating, fatigue, headaches, lack of focus, joint pain, skin issues, and inflammation in general. No certain cause for LGS can be pinpointed, though there are certain conditions that could increase its risks, like excessive alcohol consumption, poor nutrition, autoimmune disorders, infections, diabetes, and even consistent stress (Eske, 2023).

Stress

Perhaps "stress" is one of the most frequently used words in our everyday lives. It could be caused by many reasons—physical, mental, environmental, and so on.

Stress can have adverse effects on your gut health, too! Stress can be short term or long term and become chronic depending on the situation and condition. If you are facing short- or long-term stress, some of the signs you might experience are loss of appetite, gastrointestinal issues like indigestion, and stomach aches. Chronic stress can also lead to irritable bowel syndrome and many other serious GI conditions.

Maintaining a healthy diet, including prebiotics and probiotics, can help increase the good bacteria present in the gut and help ease the digestive process (Hill, 2018).

Altered Gut Bacteria

The human gut is said to contain more than 100 million microbes, comprising bacteria that are good for overall health. These good bacteria help fight the bad bacteria that can cause severe health risks and conditions. According to Dr. Friedman, if there is an alteration or imbalance in the gut bacteria and the microbiome, that can lead to several health issues, including inflammation (Godman, 2021).

Studies show that intestinal microflora plays a significant role in transmitting messages between the brain and the gut, supplying nutrients, helping in cellulose digestion, and synthesizing vitamin K. Because of this, the human microbiome is also referred to as the "second brain," and any imbalance or alteration in it caused by the use of antibiotics, stress, aging, bad dietary choices, an unhealthy lifestyle, or illnesses can lead to several conditions, including Alzheimer's disease (Dicks, 2022).

Apart from the mentioned conditions, there are a few other areas of concern that could be responsible for aggravating the risk of inflammation and diseases related to digestive disorders. For example:

- **Medications:** Medications used to curb and treat many illnesses, like anti-inflammatory medicines, antibiotics, and even oral contraceptive pills, can cause the risk of conditions like IBD.

- **Genetics:** Genetics can be blamed for increasing the risk of developing many health issues, including inflammatory bowel diseases. Due to cases of gene mutation, the immune system of the human body can be altered to a great extent and further cause issues.

- **Lifestyle and diet:** Lifestyle and diet can be huge factors influencing your health. Consistent consumption of red meat, highly processed food, saturated fat, smoking, drinking alcohol, and a life without much physical activity can lead to the risk of many health complications, such as digestive disorders, inflammation, weight gain, and even conditions of IBD (Godman, 2021).

The importance of microbes in your gut cannot be overlooked. From digesting food to improving your immunity and overall health, microbes can protect you from countless diseases. As we have already seen, an imbalance and alteration in the gut microflora can cause severe health conditions and even weight gain. We cannot ignore that there are numerous advantages of having a healthy gut microbiome to overall gut, heart, and brain health.

Navigating a Flat Belly With Food Sensitivities

A healthy lifestyle with a weight that is on par with your body mass index (BMI), body fat percentage, and muscle mass amounts can be a great feeling overall. Nonetheless, shedding a few pounds and losing a few inches around the belly can be difficult to achieve without a healthy diet and physical routine. And for those who have food allergies and food intolerance, finding the perfect diet can be quite a difficult task.

Of course, to make things easier, there are countless products available on the market that sell with "allergen-free" labels on them. These can be more convenient but can be very costly in the long run. So, why not get a few ideas that can not only help you with your weight loss journey but also help you understand how to keep a distance from foods that can make you sick?

Identifying Alternative Options and Substitutions

Maintaining a weight-reduction regimen can be complicated for those with particular food sensitivities and allergies because many of the foods advised for weight management may not be the best choice for you. The best course of action in this situation is to adhere to a few rules when choosing your meals, along with searching for alternatives and substitutions as much as you can.

Here are a few suggestions:

Consult a Nutritionist

For someone who has allergies or is prone to food intolerance, the first step is to consult with a professional dietician or a nutritionist. In today's world, there is a lot of information given on the internet regarding health conditions, which can cause more damage if false. So, having professional guidance is the best way to understand your allergies and learn methods to keep your condition in check. On the Lifelong Metabolic Center program, we utilize all-natural, anti-inflammatory, and low glycemic foods all outside of the top five food sensitivity groups. In Phase 4, we can do a "reverse elimination" process to determine potential food sensitivities before returning anything to your regular daily intake. We believe it is best to do a metabolic reset utilizing these foods and then help you find the right foods for *you* lifelong.

Keep a Food Journal

One of the most effective ways to keep yourself healthy and in good shape is to be mindful of your food choices. Taking note of the foods that tend to make you feel sick or queasy might not only help you remember the specifics but can also be extremely helpful in an emergency. Making sure to inform the chef or the restaurant staff of any ingredients or food components that you cannot have on your plate is a must every single time you eat out. However, if you feel self-conscious about it, then you can simply ask for the ingredients that have been used in your food. Staying vigilant as well as averting complications before they develop is always better than seeking a solution afterward.

Go for Food Allergy Alternatives

Some of the most common food allergens are milk, eggs, peanuts, tree nuts, shellfish, fish, and soybeans. Though these food items may not be completely replaceable in certain dishes, there are a few other alternatives you can use to still enjoy tastes similar to these.

Here are some of the most widely used food alternatives that people with food intolerance and allergy issues can opt for:

Milk Substitutes

Coconut, soy, oats, almonds, cashews, hazelnuts, rice, potato, sunflower, and macadamia milk can be used to replace cow's milk for a variety of uses. These kinds of milk are created from plant sources and are also rich in vitamins A and D. Studies show that around 80% of milk intolerance cases increase within a span of two to three years. Milk is very commonly used all around the globe.

From milk tea to puddings, there are numerous delicacies that are prepared with it (Solinas et al., 2010).

The risk of lactose intolerance highly persists for people who have food intolerance issues. In most cases, doctors advise people to avoid dairy and milk products completely, and that can be a big challenge for those who crave milk products. In such a case, milk substitutes can be a real win.

Egg Substitutes

Eggs can be a part of countless delicious dishes and are used almost everywhere in the world. They are used in batters, baking, salads, and a wide range of manufactured products as well. This can make it difficult for someone with an egg allergy to find food products without eggs. There could be chances of cross-contamination in many foods, especially while eating out in a restaurant, making it all the more difficult for allergic patients.

Eggs are widely used as binding agents when frying, baking, or cooking food. If you can't use eggs due to allergy, you can use other forms of binding substitutes while preparing your desired dish. For binding, you can use apple sauce, mashed bananas, and ground flaxseed mixed with water. Similarly, gelatin and sometimes corn flour can also be used in place of eggs for cooking purposes.

Wheat Substitutes

Wheat is one of the most common ingredients used for cooking in nearly every part of the world, but many people are also allergic to wheat. Wheat is found in a large number of food products, and it is very difficult to track whether food has been contaminated by wheat.

Celiac disease is distinct from a wheat allergy, despite seeming similar. Wheat allergy has to do with antibodies, but celiac disease is about a reaction to gluten, a type of protein present in wheat that causes immune system problems (Cianferoni, 2016).

There is a wide range of flours available on the market that are gluten and wheat free. Flours made from coconut, almond, oats, and rice are some of the most common substitutes for wheat. These flours are not only helpful in avoiding allergies and sensitivity to gluten and wheat but are also rich in nutritional value, including fiber and minerals. Almond flour, for instance, is known to help control cholesterol issues and can be used just like wheat for baking and cooking. From packaged food that is gluten free to bread and pasta that are made from buckwheat, millet, potatoes, rice, tapioca, and chickpea flour, these are some great substitutes for wheat that you can use to prepare your food.

Protein

There are many cases where people suffer from dietary protein intolerance. This is a clinical syndrome caused by the absorption of proteins through permeable mucosa in the small intestine. It is the protein in cow's milk that causes numerous children to become intolerant of it (Walker-Smith, 1988).

Protein is very important for building muscles, neurological functions, hormonal balance, and overall health. Fish and shellfish are good sources of omega-3 fatty acids and proteins, but people sensitive to and allergic to their proteins have problems consuming them. However, protein is a must in your diet, and if you cannot consume fish or seafood, you can opt for various other protein substitutes, like eggs, yogurt, grass-fed meat, and poultry. Similarly, if you choose a vegetarian diet, then plant-based proteins, like black beans, natto, and lentils, are some great options. Walnuts, chia seeds, and flaxseed are also sources of fiber, minerals, vitamins, and protein (Ruggeri, 2016).

While on a fitness journey, the food you eat does not have to be bland and taste bad. If you are allergic to animal protein, there are many plant-based protein options on the market that not only help you prepare the type of meal you want but also taste just the same! Alternatives and substitutes are always there to help you with your fitness goals and enhance your taste bud experience.

Challenges to Lose Weight With Food Allergies and Intolerance

Checking the scales every now and then can be demotivating if you do not see the result you aimed for. Belly fat is so stubborn that it takes a lot of diet control, exercise, and, most importantly, reduced stress. While these criteria may seem achievable, one thing that remains of primary concern is whether your food allergies and sensitivities are causing hurdles in the process of your weight loss.

Food is an essential part of our lives, and when it comes to health, your diet and lifestyle play a huge role. Weight loss is not just about eating less; it is about eating right. There is no doubt that counting macros is one of the best ways to shed extra weight. It is understandable that allergies and food sensitivity can cause immense discomfort and hurdles in regular life and in your efforts to work on your fitness, but that should not stop you from trying.

Tennis player Novak Djokovic, for example, is known to be gluten intolerant. Interestingly, he grew up in a household that had a pizza restaurant, which meant he was surrounded by bread, pasta, and everything gluten. It wasn't until he entirely eliminated gluten from his diet that his asthma, colds, flu, and allergies disappeared. His family was worried because he started to lose weight and lost around 11 pounds after he ditched gluten. He could, however, sense the good flow of energy and increasing stamina, and rightfully so. A few years later, he won 10 titles, 43 straight matches, three grand slams, and many more (*Is a Food Intolerance Making Weight Loss Difficult?* 2014).

This shows how determination and willpower, even amidst the biggest of temptations, can help you achieve your goals. In Novak Djokovic's case, we can see that staying in an environment with gluten around and staying away from it must have been extremely difficult. Similarly, if we try to understand our health conditions and food intolerances, we will be able to find ways to make tweaks to our diet and lifestyle and work toward achieving our goal of losing weight and some waistline inches, too!

Food Allergy and Weight Gain Connection

How can being allergic to eggs and unable to eat them lead you to gain weight? That does seem bizarre! It is true that food sensitivities and allergies have some link when it comes to the problems of losing weight.

Here are a few ways your food allergies can create some hurdles in your effort to lose weight:

Diet

When you are allergic to certain foods, like eggs, peanuts, and certain fruits, your diet becomes restricted to a few other items only. When on a weight-loss plan, having nutritious and healthy food is very important. However, with food restrictions due to allergies, numerous nutritious foods get eliminated from your regular diet. For example, by cutting eggs, milk, and peanuts from your diet, you reduce the intake of all the goodness that foods like these provide in terms of protein and nutrients. This increases the risk of an imbalance in the diet and can impact your metabolism further, making it difficult to lose weight and cut stubborn fat from the body.

Furthermore, there is a tendency to look for alternatives while shopping for allergen-free items; but, again, if you don't study the labels carefully, you could end up consuming more hidden sugar, extra calories, and unnecessary fats that could again lead to weight gain and many other health issues.

Reduced Physical Activities

Allergies can cause severe health conditions, like rashes, swelling, and itching. If not treated well, allergy symptoms can cause a huge setback in leading a regular life. It is natural to feel exhausted when you are constantly feeling dizzy, nauseated, sneezing, itching, down with the flu, and the like. When you are not in your best health, working out or even running your everyday errands can seem like a mammoth task. Imagine a situation where you have nasal congestion and itching at the same time. It would be almost impossible to even go for a walk!

Fatigue, difficulty breathing, and the anxiety caused by allergies can be reasons enough to make you feel burdened to take a step ahead and start exercising. To maintain and lose weight, along with a healthy diet, staying physically active is a must. However, if you are prone to food sensitivity and allergies, then the symptoms might make it more of a challenge to stick to a workout regimen and strive to get in better shape.

Emotional Eating

Consider falling sick because of some food allergy, and to top it all, refrain from eating something you find delicious and lip-smackingly good! Every time you crave something, instead of simply placing an order and eating, you have to go through the pain of checking with the restaurant about the ingredients and the labels on the food. It can be a tiring process and enough reason to feel frustrated and exhausted in the long run.

Just like binge-watching a TV series is a way to kill boredom, so is emotional eating a way to cope with the frustration of constant allergies that are a hindrance to leading a normal life. Staying at home and binging on food in an effort to feel better can be a great way to escape reality for some time. However, in that process, emotional eating increases your calorie intake and can be enough to make you gain weight in the long run.

Food allergies can impact many other aspects of your life, not just your health. For instance, socializing with friends and family may seem like a task because of not being able to participate and freely eat anything from the plate. Food is an essential part of gatherings and is also a medium through which people bond. Being unable to eat out freely can adversely affect your social relationships and even your self-esteem.

Habit replacement is a great thing to work toward if you are an emotional eater. When you crave food and eat that food, you are getting an internal shot of dopamine. This is the "high" you feel from emotional eating. If you replace the habit with a healthier habit that gives you the same high (shot of dopamine), then you end up with a comparable coping mechanism that has a healthier outcome. Try cleaning out a cabinet, painting your nails, calling a friend, doing jumping jacks, or anything that sounds fun to you and takes about the same amount of time as eating a snack, about three to five minutes. Make a list of these and go to your list the next time you want to eat due to emotion rather than hunger.

Medications

One of the most common medications given for allergic reactions is called antihistamine. Medicines like Allegra, Benadryl, Claritin, and Zyrtec are some of the antihistamines used all over the globe to counter allergic reactions. These medications are highly effective and powerful, but they also have a few adverse effects, like weight gain.

In some of the medicines prescribed by doctors, there is a substantial quantity of steroids, which can manage symptoms caused by allergic responses but can also make losing weight a bit difficult. Also, most antihistamine medicines are known to create a drowsy feeling and act as an effective sedative. The heaviness and sleepy feeling can make it very difficult for you to go out for physical activity, yet regular workouts are necessary to burn calories and achieve optimal health.

So, losing weight while dealing with allergies can be a difficult task. However, with a little more awareness, conscious eating, and regular exercise, you can deal with these issues and strive to achieve your best health and fitness. Choose from foods you have no allergy or sensitivity to in order to get closer to the flat belly you.

Chapter 5:

Prioritizing Bowel

Regularity

Time to talk poop! Probably got a giggle out of you, but it's a little talked about topic, and we gotta hit it here when addressing flat belly goals. Bowel movements are absolutely important for your general health.

When this topic pops up, it's cringy for many of us, and we would rather push even the slightest conversations mentioning "poop" aside. First, no worries, because it is a very natural process and has to be equally paid attention to as we would for the rest of our bodily functions. So, bowel movements must be understood and carefully studied for greater awareness of how they affect how we live our lives for maximum vitality.

Understanding the Importance of Regular Bowel Movements

We don't waste a minute appreciating our lungs and respiratory system for the air we are able to breathe (especially if you have been sick and congested or struggled to breathe recently), and very rightly so because that keeps us living. However, if I start thanking my regular bowel movements for keeping me healthy, I bet everyone will be rather shocked and maybe disgusted as well. LOL! Our holistic health depends on various factors, and to feel healthy and fit, every organ and aspect of our systems should function at peak levels. But I am not exaggerating here: Regular bowel movements are vital for overall health and definitely for a flat stomach.

So, what is considered a regular healthy bowel movement? This can have various answers, as the frequency of bowel movements is not the same for everyone. For example, some may have bowel movements every day and, sometimes, even twice a day. For some, it might be an occurrence only three times or once a week. So, according to your unique bowel patterns, you can understand what falls within your general norms.

Here are some of the reasons why regular bowel movements are necessary:

- **Removing of waste:** Simply put, bowel movements help the system to empty the intestine and get rid of the waste and toxins present. It is a very integral process for human health. It flushes out the toxins and harmful substances from the colon.

- **Preventing diseases:** Irregular bowel movements can cause severe discomfort, the formation of gas, bloating, and constipation issues. These issues can further lay the groundwork for several other diseases, like colorectal issues, hemorrhoids, abdominal pain, a weakened immune system, and, in some cases, cancer. Difficulty passing stool regularly can also cause rectal bleeding, anal fissures, nausea, and excessive pain. However, regular bowel movements can help prevent such conditions.

From toxin removal to improving the quality of life, regular and healthy-sized or shaped bowel movements can be extremely beneficial for your wellness.

Role in Digestive Health and Flat Belly Goals

Your bowel movement patterns say a lot about your digestive and gut health. Regular and smooth passing indicates that the food consumed is well broken down in the system, the nutrients are well absorbed in the body, and the gut feels healthy due to the presence of good microbes, making your immunity strong. In addition, this can be advantageous for those trying to maintain their weight and, in many cases, lose some weight as well.

An interesting study shows how your bowel can give a clear insight into why you are not able to lose belly fat! A study was done on the bacterial diversity of 3,600 bowel samples from 1,300 twins. Their visceral body fat and subcutaneous fat were measured, and the result found through comparison was that the more diverse and variant their microbiome was, the lower their risk of getting obese and having visceral fat (Mackenzie, 2016). Through this research, we see that your gut health is directly responsible for helping maintain weight. While one study may not be definitive, there is definitely no harm in giving it some importance and taking good care by eating right.

One question that instantly pops up in this case is: Does your bowel movement really affect your weight-loss effort? The answer can be a bit complex. There are many people who experience a drop in their weight after a bout of vomiting and diarrhea. To be precise, if you check your weight after a day or two of having diarrhea, the drop in weight that you see on the scale is all about the water weight and not at all about any permanent fat loss. The two types of fat we have in our bodies are visceral and subcutaneous fat. The former is the fat that is gathered around your organs, and thus in the waist, and can be very dangerous for overall health, and the latter is mostly the fat that is beneath the skin (Walters, 2018).

As we have already discussed in the previous chapters, sticking to macro counting and maintaining a healthy lifestyle with regular exercise are the most effective ways to reduce fat and lose weight. A healthy colon with no gas or waste stuck can make the belly appear and feel flat. However, with constipation and digestive issues, you can feel bloated, which is why regular bowel movement is so important. Having said that, it is true that regular bowel movements can help you stay comfortable and even feel light, but losing weight by pooping a lot quickly really does not make any sense for a long-term weight-loss and weight-maintenance strategy.

Signs of Healthy Bowel Function

Two of the indicators for understanding healthy bowel function are its consistency and color.

Stool Color

The color, texture, and consistency of your stool can depend on various simple factors, like the type of food you ate the day before or the amount of fluids you drank. There could be many underlying causes for a certain abnormality if it stays the same for a prolonged period. However, the color of your stool can say a lot about your health.

- **Brown:** All brown-colored stools are considered normal. The bile formed in the liver mixes with the digested food in the intestine, which results in a brown color.

- **Yellow:** A yellow-colored stool with a slight odor and grease could indicate some bacterial infections and digestive issues. It is mainly seen in babies who breastfeed.

- **Green:** Green stool could be caused by medications, like iron supplements and antibiotics. Consumption of green vegetables and drinks could also be the reason for the color. It could be caused by particular foods or drinks that passed through the gut and did not digest well, indicating a gastrointestinal disorder as well.

- **Red:** It is usually the food and drinks you consume that can cause red stool. However, if the stool is consistently red, then that could be because of some bleeding in the gastrointestinal tract.

- **Black:** A few medicines, like iron supplements, can cause the stool to turn black. Similarly, certain foods, like blueberries, blood sausages, black licorice, etc., can cause the same. However, if there is no such food consumed, it could hint at an underlying condition, like bleeding in the intestines.

If you notice that you are consistently getting such colored stool without consuming any food or drinks that could possibly cause it, you should visit your doctor for a thorough checkup (Alzayer, 2022).

Stool Consistency

Regular bowel movements indicate good gastrointestinal health. Irregular bowel movements, at times, do not pose any immediate harm; but if continued for a prolonged amount of time, it can be problematic.

According to the Bristol stool chart, there are seven different types of stool consistency, and each could indicate a certain condition. Let us look at them in detail:

- **Type 1:** This type of stool is hard, separate, and, in the form of lumps, feels like constipation and can be quite difficult to pass.

- **Type 2:** This type of stool looks like sausage but is a bit lumpy. It could indicate that you are constipated.

- **Type 3:** This type of stool also looks like sausage, but it has cracks on the surface area.

- **Type 4:** This type of stool also looks like sausage but is very soft and smooth.

- **Type 5:** This type of stool has clear-cut edges and is in the form of soft blobs, which are very easy to pass.

- **Type 6:** This type of stool is mushy, fluffy in texture, and very easy to pass.

- **Type 7:** This type of stool is entirely in liquid form.

Dr. Ken Heaton, assisted by 66 volunteers from the University of Bristol, generated this chart in 1997 (WebMD Editorial Contributors, 2015). There has been remarkable documented information that has helped in understanding the complexities of health with regard to the bowel style and movements of a person.

Factors Influencing Bowel Regularity

Bowel movements and their regularity vary from person to person. If you have watched *The Big Bang Theory*, you know that it is a fantastic sitcom where the lead character

Sheldon is a scientist and is extremely particular about his bathroom schedule. He is a genius who insists on keeping this bathroom schedule because it is true: Your habits and routines play a major role in deciding at what time and how frequently you will poop. Although a little nutty, he wasn't wrong!

Many factors contribute to frequent or fewer bowel movements. Here are a few primary factors influencing bowel regularity:

Dietary Fiber and Hydration

Studies show that around 27% of adults suffer from symptoms of constipation, bloating, gas, and digestion-related conditions caused mainly by increasing age and a more sedentary lifestyle (Petre, 2017).

The foods you consume play a key role in how your bowel movement will be. Dietary fiber is an integral part of a well-rounded diet. It is great for accelerating bowel movements and also helps prevent constipation problems. Dietary fibers are divided into two categories:

- **Insoluble fiber:** This type of fiber accelerates the frequency and bulk of stool.

- **Soluble fiber:** This type of fiber helps regulate blood sugar and cholesterol levels.

Eating fiber-rich food can significantly help in regulating bowel movements. Drinking enough water and keeping your body hydrated at all times is also vital. Water helps digest food, makes the stool softer, and prevents the risk of constipation.

Lifestyle Habits and Stress Management

Your dietary lifestyle habits have an impact on your social life, job, health, and happiness in general. The condition of your digestive system is impacted by the food you eat, your physical exertion level, and your degree of stress, which might result in bowel habits that are inconsistent.

If you are facing issues with digestive health and bowel movement issues, you should make an effort to stay away from the following:

- **Red meat:** Red meat contains proteins and several micronutrients, but it is extremely low in fiber. This is one of the reasons why the consumption of red meat in excess can increase the risk of severe constipation. It is heavy for your system, can cause bulkiness in the stool, and can cause irregular bowel movements. By making a conscious effort, you can opt for plant-based protein sources, like lentils, legumes, beans, etc., instead of devouring a heavy steak if it is causing bowel issues for you.

- **Alcohol:** Drinking an excessive amount of alcohol can lead to dehydration, which can further cause severe health conditions. With dehydration, the risk of constipation increases as the frequency of urination also slows down. However, the effects of alcohol can have different consequences for different people. For example, in many cases, after drinking for the whole night or in large quantities, some may even get stomach upset and diarrhea.

- **Dairy products:** Studies were done by replacing cow's milk with soy milk and giving it to children suffering from chronic constipation. It was seen that cow's milk aggravated their constipation, and when the milk was changed to soy milk, their condition improved, and they got relief. The protein found in cow's milk can cause mild to severe complications if you have digestive and food intolerance issues (Crowley et al., 2008).

- **Processed grains:** Flour used in pasta, white bread, and noodles is mostly processed and contains very little fiber, which can cause constipation and other digestive issues. This is one of the reasons why nutritionists often suggest whole grains as an alternative to processed grains, where the bran and fiber present in the grains are removed during processing. Fiber helps in bowel movement, but again, it depends on the health and condition of the patient.

- **Gluten:** There are many who are intolerant to gluten, which is a protein found in grains like barley, wheat, rye, triticale, and kamut. Especially for a person suffering from celiac disease, consumption of gluten-laden food can cause more intolerance issues and inflame their immune system. Chronic constipation is another adverse effect that could result from consumption of gluten.

- **Stress:** Studies show how stress can adversely affect a person's overall health, including digestive and bowel movement dysfunction. When a person faces stress, their body releases a hormone called epinephrine as a response. This diverts the blood flow to other organs from the intestine, and the intestinal movement slows down, causing constipation. The permeability of the intestine also increases, causing a feeling of fullness and discomfort in the abdomen (Petre, 2020).

In some cases, people do not even realize that the food and drinks they are consuming cause bowel-related problems. With the increase in access to takeout and fast food joints, we, as a society, are consuming more processed food without even realizing it. For example, in the case of mass-baked brown bread, some buy it thinking there is no flour in it. This could be a serious concern for those struggling with gluten allergies, because if you check the label, you will notice that there is white flour in it, which, in my opinion, makes brown bread lose its purpose. Your lifestyle plays a huge role in how you feel physically and mentally. More so, if you have food intolerance and allergy issues, you must all the more be aware of what you consume. Reading the labels on food items and being aware of what makes your bowel regular can also help you feel better in the long run, in addition to helping keep your stomach from protruding.

Practical Strategies for Improving Bowel Regularity

Diet Modifications and Hydration Practices

Sometimes, health issues are such that regardless of how much you try, you may not be able to avoid them altogether. The best you can do is find ways to keep them at bay as much as possible. Imagine reaching an age where it becomes extremely difficult to reverse many ailments and diseases. To prevent that from happening, efforts must be made *now* to make dietary modifications and increase hydration, along with adopting a healthy lifestyle.

Here are a few tips that can help you do it in an easy way:

Increase Fiber-Rich Foods in Your Diet

Americans are said to consume quite less than the recommended daily dose of fiber, which for women is 25 grams and for men is 38 grams per day. Beans, broccoli, berries, avocados, whole grains, popcorn, lentils, chia seeds, dried fruits, apples, nuts, potatoes, split peas, chickpeas, quinoa, almonds, pears, oats, bananas, carrots, beets, artichoke, Brussels sprouts, kale, spinach, tomatoes, sweet potatoes, dark chocolates, etc., are some of the sources of fiber. However, it has to be noted that increasing fiber in your diet quickly is not recommended. You should gradually introduce or increase the portion of fiber-rich foods in your diet. The correct amount of fiber intake can help with weight loss, diabetes, and improving bowel movements (Gunnars, 2020).

Include Probiotics in Your Diet

As we know, gut health and its microbiome have a major role to play in keeping the gastrointestinal tract and digestive health healthy and functioning. The good bacteria in your system not only help improve immunity but also improve digestive functions, making bowel movements smooth, too. A healthy gut also helps you maintain and lose weight by increasing your metabolism as a whole. Lifelong Metabolic Center has a fantastic probiotic available over the counter. Look for a USP label to ensure probiotics have been quality tested by a third party that had nothing to gain from the outcome of the testing.

Check for Food Sensitivity

Food sensitivity is one of the many reasons for getting bowel issues like constipation. For example, when milk protein is not digested well in the system, it causes flatulence, diarrhea, or even constipation. Eliminate or replace any food item that causes you discomfort and digestion issues. Using excessive oil while cooking or having too many dairy products can affect your health in the long run or give *you* the runs in the short run.

Avoid Processed Food

Most processed foods contain high levels of sodium, flour, preservatives, and artificial colors and are generally very low in fiber. Consuming processed food in excess can cause many health issues, like constipation, high cholesterol, and blood pressure issues. Regular intake of such food can heavily affect your metabolism and cause weight gain.

Eat Prunes

Prunes are rich in polyphenols, fructans, fiber, probiotics, and sorbitol. They are exceptionally good for bowel movements. They have laxative properties and are said to relieve constipation and also help regulate stool volume and frequency of bowel movements. But again, don't overdo these, or you can end up with gas and/or diarrhea.

A Few Herbs and Tips That Help

There are numerous natural treatments and supplements available to help reduce conditions of bowel movements, like diarrhea, constipation, and many other digestive issues.

For diarrhea

- Bovine colostrum is the milk produced immediately and for a few days after a cow gives birth. It is rich in antibodies, cytokines, and growth factors, which help treat diarrhea in adults.

- Berberine is a medicinal plant with microbial properties that helps fight viruses, fungi, and bacteria and also helps with diarrhea.

- Similarly, chamomile and berry leaf teas are beneficial in reducing inflammation in the gut. Ginger can help with diarrhea caused by IBS.

For constipation

- Senna tea is a traditional herb used to clean the colon.

- Cascara sagrada falls under unregulated herbal supplements but has been used over the years for relieving constipation.

- Amalaka powder is used in Ayurvedic medicine, is beneficial for digestion, and is said to ease constipation as well.

- Triphala is also an herb used in Ayurvedic medicine and is said to have a laxative effect. It can help reduce bloating, abdominal pain, and bowel issues.

- Peppermint oil can be great for digestive health. It relaxes the gut muscles and reduces abdominal pain.

- Artichoke leaf extract is very effective in regulating bowel issues, especially constipation problems.

- Aloe vera is a plant that helps to reduce the effects of IBS, diabetes, constipation, and many skin issues as well.

- Slippery elm is an herbal medicine that has been used by Native Americans to treat many health issues. It has a calming effect on the intestines and eases diarrhea or constipation.

For dehydration

Bowel issues like constipation can be caused by dehydration. Many times, when the food you consume lacks water content, the large intestine will make an effort to pull water from the waste instead. This can cause hard stool and constipation issues, further causing pain during bowel movements

Drinking more water and eating foods with a high water content can help prevent dehydration. Your body loses a lot of water during and after strenuous physical activities, like exercise and even walking daily, especially on hot days. Through sweat and urine, the body loses water, and if not replenished with more water intake, there can be serious dehydration issues.

Drink half of your body weight in ounces per day. Drink enough water and avoid caffeinated drinks. If the dehydration is a bit more than normal, then having fluids with electrolytes can be very helpful as well. Gatorade has recently come out with some lighter versions with less sugar and all-natural ingredients. You can even boil a banana with the ends cut off and drink the "tea" to get your electrolytes back in check as well.

Incorporating Physical Activity and Stress-Reduction Techniques

Stress is a part of modern-day existence. There are so many factors that you deal with every single day of your life that can impact your mind and health in many different ways. When your body and mind are not in sync, stress can take over your holistic wellness.

Physical activities play a significant role in managing stress. This happens because when your body is physically active and moving, blood circulation increases, which positively affects your brain health. Endorphins, also referred to as "feel-good hormones," help reduce stress and give a positive "high" after physical activity, which is one of the primary reasons why most people feel happy after a good workout.

By incorporating regular exercises and a few stress-reduction methods, you can regulate many health conditions—including bowel irregularities.

Here are a few benefits exercises can bring:

- Studies show that regular exercise can enhance your immunity, reduce inflammation, and decrease the risk of getting several diseases. With exercise, blood and lymph flow increase and so does your immune cell circulation.

- Regular exercise helps reduce the risk of cardiovascular diseases and even bone health conditions.

- Physical activities can cause a slight alteration in antibodies and white blood cells, which are the immune system cells of the body that help fight against diseases.

- With regular workouts and physical activities, bacteria are flushed out of the system through the airways, which helps prevent flu-type symptoms/conditions.

- After physical activity, body temperature slightly increases, which is said to prevent the spread of bacteria and infections, similar to how fever fights against infections.

- Stress can cause severe illnesses, but with regular exercise, the production of cortisol, a stress hormone, decreases, resulting in a lowered risk of ailments caused by stress. There are direct correlations between a reduction in cortisol and a reduction in belly fat, too.

- Exercise can make you feel better and happier! Physical activities help produce endorphins, the hormones responsible for reducing pain and inducing happiness. This is one of the reasons why after a good workout, you feel uplifted and positive.

- A study showed how regular exercise for about six weeks can reduce tiredness for people who reportedly complained about fatigue for a very long time (Loy et al., 2013). This shows how regular exercise can help increase your energy levels.

- Regular exercise is said to reduce hypertension and can also reduce the risk of developing cardiovascular conditions.

- Exercise is effective in reducing constipation and regulating bowel movements. With exercises like aerobics and cardio, your heart and breathing rate increase because the contraction of muscles in the intestine is increased making it easier to help excrete stools easily (Fulghum, 2007).

- Exercising and keeping yourself physically active throughout the day can help you sleep better at night.

I understand that working out at a gym or going out for a run may not be always feasible. However, the key is moving your body as much as you can! Regardless of how busy your schedule is or where you are, ensure that you give yourself a minimum of 20 to 30 minutes each day to do some stretches, on-the-spot jogging, yoga poses, or any convenient exercise. Inactivity is a major culprit for weight gain, and if it is combined with excessive stress and exhaustion, it becomes especially problematic for your belly fat as well.

The American Heart Association recommends a minimum of 150 minutes of moderate exercise a week. Being physically active can divert your attention from stressful thoughts and situations and make you feel better and more positive. The more physically active you are, the more connected you will feel to the rhythm of your body and movements. Exercising can not only make you physically fit but can also keep your mind calm and relaxed.

Exercises like biking, hiking, brisk walking, jogging, swimming, climbing stairs, water aerobics, dancing, rowing, playing a sport, and other forms of aerobic exercise are extremely beneficial in managing stress, improving health, and reducing weight. If you ever feel anxious or if anger is bubbling up inside of you, try taking a quiet walk outside. In no time, you will sense how your stress fades, and you will feel energetic and much happier (Madel, 2012).

Tips to Reduce Stress in General

When we are young, we don't have to think much about taking care of ourselves. Our bodies are strong and energetic. With growing age and added responsibilities in life, our physical and mental health tend to take a back seat to the hustle and bustle of middle-aged lifestyles. Slowly, stress and exhaustion creep in and often leave behind several health complications before we realize it. We don't feel old mentally, but we start to *feel* old physically long before we should. If we start to pay attention *now* and take action *now*, we can stretch our vitality much, much longer.

This is one of the reasons why anyone, regardless of age, can and should start a self-care routine and attempt every approach to reduce stress in any form. We all know by now how excessive stress can cause health issues and can lead to many bowel issues as well.

Here are a few tips that can guide you to help reduce stress:

- **Exercise regularly:** Regular activities can keep your mind stress free and happy. The hormones produced after your body goes through a workout can make you feel happy and relieve stress and anxiety.

- **Follow a diet plan:** A well-rounded diet free from processed and artificial foods can add more benefits to your health and keep your body and mind clean and healthy. Stress and anxiety can cause many hindrances to your diet routine. For example, cases like binge eating or eating less due to stress can cause severe nutrient deficiency and, in many cases, bloating and weight gain or loss issues. Following a healthy diet plan is essential for staying low stress.

- **Reduce screen time:** Excessive use of gadgets can cause anxiety, frustration, and low psychological well-being. By reducing screen time, you can get more time for yourself and sleep better at night, too.

- **Remember self-care:** Prioritizing your health and well-being is the best way to detox and de-stress your mind and body. Make time for yourself and try activities you enjoy. For example, read a book, light scented candles, take a relaxing bath, get a massage, take a walk, practice yoga, or do something that works for you and makes you feel refreshed, renewed, and restored.

- **Journal:** It is normal to feel the desire to let your emotions and anxieties out when you are overwhelmed and overloaded. It might not always be feasible or even the best course of action. So, keeping a journal can be a great outlet. Before going to bed, you might write about how your mental and physical health has changed over the day. By doing this, you will feel less stressed and will be able to subsequently identify all of your behavioral patterns and discover appropriate potential solutions.

- **Limit caffeine and alcohol:** The caffeine present in coffee, chocolate, tea, and energy drinks is known to stimulate your brain. Excessive consumption of caffeine can cause anxiety and can also cause insomnia. Cutting back on such caffeinated drinks and switching to drinking more water and herbal teas can be a better option to help reduce stress. Similarly, reducing the intake of alcohol can also help in reducing stress and anxiety.

- **Surround yourself with loved ones:** One study showed how young adults tend to suffer from depression, loneliness, and stress symptoms when they receive very little or no support from their friends, family, and partners (Lee et al., 2020). Spending time and doing things that you love with those you love (and like being around) can uplift your mood and fill your spirit with positivity and happiness. This can be an effective way to curb stress and anxiety.

- **Avoid procrastination:** Without a doubt, overthinking is a cause of stress, but more than that, a habit of procrastination can be a problematic issue that can cause stress, too. For example, when you decide to do something later, the thought of doing it and completing it will keep circling your mind, and eventually, the more you extend, the longer you will feel stressed about it. Avoiding procrastination decreases the amount of time that task is draining your mental energy.

- **Learn to say "no":** The burden of doing something when you don't want to or feel up for it can be negative for your mind. The stress you get from saying "yes" to someone or something when you don't mean it or want it can make you restless and frustrated. Saying a clear "no" to things you do not want can clear your headspace and also help you feel better and less responsible for anything not needed in your life.

- **Try yoga:** A great way to counter stress is by practicing yoga, the age-old form of exercise known for its benefits for your holistic health. There are different poses and asanas in yoga for every body part and a variety of health conditions. I even started doing face yoga recently. It is an amazing way to drain lymph in your face, neck, and shoulders; increase circulation; and perhaps even avoid a wrinkle or two. The jury is still out on that one. Check back with me in a few years, and we will see. From relieving body aches and losing weight to healing the body and calming the mind, yoga can boost your health and well-being.

- **Meditate:** Mindful meditation has been practiced by people for thousands of years. The benefits of meditation, especially mindful meditation, can help your mind in many ways. It can balance your mind and body and sync them so beautifully that your body becomes less stressed and healthier over time.

- **Go outside:** Nature is the ultimate healer! Studies show how spending even as little as 10 minutes in nature can help your physical and mental well-being (Meredith et al., 2020). Taking some time out and spending it in the outdoors can not only help you feel better, but it can also give you a whole new perspective. It helps to enjoy the environment around you and appreciate the beauty of nature.

- **Engage in touch:** Having positive contact with someone, particularly physically, like a long hug or cuddle, can help soothe your mind and reduce stress. Human touch is said to be very healing and has a relieving effect of calming your mind and body. This is primarily caused by the production of oxytocin, which helps lower the stress hormone cortisol, which, in turn, has many health benefits.

- **Breathe:** Stress can cause severe changes in your mental and physical condition. The human body responds to stress and gets into a fight-or-flight mode to cope with it. An increase in stress and cortisol levels can lead to health conditions like heart palpitations, constricted blood vessels, and fast breathing. The way we breathe has a lot to do with how our bodies function. Through awareness and careful practice of different types of breathing exercises, you can feel more relaxed and rejuvenated. Some effective breathing exercises are diaphragmatic, alternate nostril, paced, and box breathing. When you are aware of your breath, you will feel more alive and conscious of the present, which will help divert your mind from stressful thoughts. Take slow and deep breaths and feel the air enter your system through your nose. Gradually fill your lungs, and when your lungs and belly fully expand, release the air slowly through your mouth. This can be one of the easiest and fastest ways to feel calm and relaxed.

- **Ask for help:** Asking for help is the bravest thing you can do! Too often, people keep their tension and worries to themselves and then face unnecessary struggles. The stress caused by mental health issues can be huge, so it is very important to acknowledge the existence of any mental health issues you are facing. Sometimes, we need help dealing with our own struggles, and sometimes we need to know how to best help those around us cope without absorbing it ourselves. Instead of being embarrassed, take the help of the people you are close to and also seek professional help if and when needed. Therapy and counseling sessions can help you understand what you are dealing with and, in turn, help you find what you need.

Conclusion

As we near the end of our journey together, it seems plausible to say that with knowledge, purpose, and the will to make a few healthy changes, you are capable of accomplishing unimaginably great things! Through this book, I embarked on a mission to reach out to those who have had doubts about their fitness and overall well-being and are searching for some great tips and tricks to achieve a flat(er) belly. The way our bodies act and react is something we hardly sit and think about in this era of hustle and bustle. I'm sure you would agree with me when I say that our health has taken a big hit from living this way—too fast and too furious.

A sedentary lifestyle, which is commonplace for many, has increased the risk of several health concerns, including problems with unhealthy weight and weight gain. Though everyone *can* work to achieve and maintain the size they want, it isn't always easy. It is also true that the larger your waistline, the higher the chances of disease. Everything we do is associated in some way or another with how we feel. It is not about reaching for stereotypical beauty standards by encouraging you to shed a few inches from your waist; it is about awareness of health and fitness that makes me say that it is better to work and sweat now and lose those inches than face problems due to lack of vitality later in life.

Summing Up the Journey

From the start of this book, the guiding aspects have focused on five factors for fighting belly flab. If we look back at the journey we have made together since way back on page 1, you will notice that the concept of weight loss is not simply about decreasing the numbers on the scale; it is about how healthy your mind and body are and the quality of life through your later years as well.

We started off discussing the salt we consume and how to avoid it or get the right amount for you, and then we gradually moved to topics like embracing healthy fats in your diet, managing gaseous food, avoiding food sensitivities, and achieving regular bowel movements. Losing belly fat was not the only focus; we discussed more about all the underlying factors you may need to address first.

In addition to demonstrating how to get a flat belly, I have tried to paint a clearer picture of the whys and hows behind each tip. Spot reduction of weight or fat is quite difficult, if not impossible, so when focusing on reducing belly fat, you must also make an effort to adopt a healthy lifestyle with a dedication to consistent dietary changes and regular movement.

Key Takeaways

Here are our Five Fast Flat Belly Facts in a nutshell:

Sodium Sensitivity

We have learned about the various aspects of sodium sensitivity and its impact on our lives. Now, you'll be better able to address your water retention difficulties. Next time you weigh yourself and see the scale jump up, do not fret! Double-check if it could be due to sodium; don't assume you need a whole new diet plan. A root-cause analysis of any issue is critical since it can avert a plethora of unnecessary concerns and worries.

Sodium sensitivity can jeopardize your overall wellness, possibly causing hypertension, cardiovascular conditions, and even stroke. Your effort to shed inches from your waist may be going well, but without realizing it, the added salt you sprinkle on your foods every time you eat could be stopping you from getting in the shape you want as quickly as you want.

Constant feelings of being bloated and puffy are not pleasant, and once you understand that it might be sodium causing these symptoms, you can take measures and make necessary lifestyle and diet changes. Often, it's enough to monitor your salt intake to address water retention issues and other ailments. However, overdoing anything may be harmful, so instead of eliminating salt completely, limit your intake to a minimum. With conscious decisions like this, you will soon see a difference in your health and weight.

Embracing Healthy Fats

While there is a widespread fear of "fat" in the world around us, don't forget that "good fats" can do wonders for your overall health! Fats are essential for your body to function at an optimal level. It helps regulate cholesterol levels, reduces inflammation, optimizes cognitive abilities, improves liver health, strengthens bones, improves skin condition, reduces sleep issues, regulates blood sugar levels, and even helps maintain weight.

If your main goal is to lose extra weight, then—contrary to what some people believe—consuming healthy fats can be advantageous. Science shows that a decent amount of healthy monosaturated fats in your daily diet can make weight loss much easier. A high-fat diet to reduce weight can work great for those who need more fats in their balanced diet, too. The Lifelong Metabolic Center Program offers a custom macro count with a simple cheek swab to tell you the exact right amount of fats for your specific body. Contact us if you are interested in losing weight or just seeing the right amounts of food and exercise for *you*.

A lack of knowledge can create countless misconceptions. Don't deprive yourself of good fats thinking that all fats are the same! You need the right information to take care of your health and wellness properly.

For example, I remember the days when I would feel bloated and, in fact, even gain substantial fat around my waist and thighs. My first reaction would be to panic, and

I would cater to all the wrong but quick fixes to solve this problem. Little did I realize that tossing out the nutritious almond butter jar in an attempt to lose weight would be one of the worst choices I made! If I had gotten the appropriate advice from an expert when I was growing up or in my teens, I would have known how to boost my body acceptance and keep active without giving up the foods I actually loved eating. The bottom line is that you don't have to give up on fats to shed fat from your body! Regardless of your age, being consistent with good, sensible choices will keep you strong and help you achieve the life you have envisioned for yourself long term.

The Buzz on Bloat

Coming back to the smelly topic of gas and gaseous food, one thing that stands out is recognizing the most common food items that tend to fill you up with gas and cause several painful side effects along with it. Gas and acidity issues can create a lot of hurdles in your everyday life. Consider the following scenario: You have a long flight with friends, and you start feeling gassy and bloated from the night before. And, to top it all off, you are freaking out you won't be *able* to hold it all in (like the poor dude on the news lately who had diarrhea and the flight had to land)! These scenarios can be avoided if you know which foods cause you distress from your food journaling.

There could be days when an antacid pill or Beano could do the trick and make you feel better in a jiffy. There could also be days when it takes exceptionally long for the gas to pass through your system, causing excessive discomfort and pain. Managing gaseous food can be tricky but is definitely not rocket science. With the help of this book, you can learn more about the digestive processes and also easily identify the various food items that could cause flatulence and chronic gas. I've mentioned in detail the different medical issues associated with gastrointestinal disorders and the various ways to prevent gas formation. With a careful selection of food and drinks, you can manage gas issues in very simple ways. Avoiding gaseous foods is an easy way to get a flatter stomach.

Food Sensitivities and Such

While it might be obvious to avoid a food you are allergic to because it gives you a rash, swelling, or difficulty breathing, sometimes figuring out food sensitivities can be much more elusive. A great way to test for these is a reverse elimination diet. By avoiding foods you are sensitive to, you can stop unnecessary belly bloat.

Poop Power

Finally, as gross as it may sound, we fixated quite a bit on bowel movements. The sensitivity around the entire "poop" discussion is real, and people prefer to not mention it, let alone discuss it out in the open. Here, I have made an effort to understand bowel movements in the most normal way, like the way we would discuss our respiratory or nervous systems. One of my goals is to create maximum awareness among my patients and followers—regardless of age, gender, or body size—to come forward and learn about their bodies.

The nature of bowel movements plays a major role in our physical and also our mental health. The food we eat and the way it gets processed and digested in the system are imperative for providing nutrients and energy throughout the body. Irregularity and difficulty in bowel movements can adversely affect your general well-being, including your mood!

Parting Wisdom

Our journey to health and happiness includes fresh knowledge, old experiences, wisdom, obstacles, and a myriad of treasures because of our years of life. When we look in the mirror, we may just see a double chin, some gray hair strands, or perhaps a button on the midriff of our shirts that has loosened due to an increasing belly. Try to also see the beautiful, amazing machine that is your body. Appreciate your abilities and gifts, too.

Whether your goal is to lose weight and flatten your stomach, to look the best you've ever looked, or to feel the healthiest you've ever felt, one thing to remember is that having the correct understanding of our physical and mental health definitely helps. Especially in this age of widely available, yet not always correct, information. From learning the effects of consuming sodium and increasing your intake of healthy fats to understanding your relationship with various food items, the way a simple nut can make you look like a puffer fish, adopting a healthy lifestyle, and understanding the true nature of your poop, we have covered it all, and I hope this knowledge will help you navigate your health issues and maybe gave you an extra smile or two here or there along the way.

Through this book, I hope you will realize the importance of being your healthiest self. Additionally, every time you think about working toward a flatter belly, may it be to feel and become as healthy as you can be. The point is not to get a large amount of "likes" and validation from social media or acceptance from your critics. Rather, it is all about loving yourself, being grateful for the health and vitality you have, and simply making the best effort to stay healthy for the longest period of time. The work you put in now can give you more years in your life and life in your years!

References

Alzayer, G. (2022, May 27). *What healthy bowel movements look like, and when to call the doctor.* Medstar Health. https://www.medstarhealth.org/blog/healthy-bowel-movements-look-like

Ball, J. (2022, August 13). *7 ways to add 10 grams of healthy fat to your meals.* Eating Well. https://www.eatingwell.com/article/7993588/ways-to-add-healthy-fat-to-your-meals/

Berry, J. (2020, January 20). *18 ways to reduce bloating: Quick tips and long-term relief.* Medical News Today. https://www.medicalnewstoday.com/articles/322525

Brehm, B. J., Lattin, B. L., Summer, S. S., Boback, J. A., Gilchrist, G. M., Jandacek, R. J., & D'Alessio, D. A. (2008). *One-year comparison of a high-monounsaturated fat diet with a high-carbohydrate diet in type 2 diabetes.* Diabetes Care, *32*(2), 215–220. https://doi.org/10.2337/dc08-0687

Cianferoni, A. (2016). *Wheat allergy: diagnosis and management.* Journal of Asthma and Allergy, 13. https://doi.org/10.2147/jaa.s81550

Cording, J. (2018, December 9). *Want to avoid gas & bloating at holiday parties? Don't eat this food.* MBG Food. https://www.mindbodygreen.com/articles/ho

w-cruciferous-vegetables-can-cause-gas-and-bloating

Crowley, E., Williams, L., Roberts, T., Jones, P., & Dunstan, R. (2008). Evidence for a role of cow's milk consumption in chronic functional constipation in children: Systematic review of the literature from 1980 to 2006. *Nutrition & Dietetics*, *65*(1), 29–35. https://doi.org/10.1111/j.1747-0080.2007.00225.x

Dallas, M. E. (2023, April 7). *Home remedies to relieve gas and reduce bloating.* EverydayHealth. https://www.everydayhealth.com/excessive-gas/home-remedies-for-gas

Dicks, L. (2022). Gut bacteria and neurotransmitters. *Microorganisms*, *10*(9), 1838. https://doi.org/10.3390/microorganisms10091838

DiLonardo, M. (2018). *Gastroenteritis (stomach "flu").* WebMD. https://www.webmd.com/digestive-disorders/gastroenteritis

Do allergies affect your gastro health? (2023, May 11). GI Associates & Endoscopy Center. https://gi.md/resources/articles/do-allergies-affect-your-gastro-health#

Dolan, E. W. (2023, June 4). *New research indicates visceral fat has a profoundly negative effect on cognitive abilities.* PsyPost. https://www.psypost.org/2023/06/new-research-indicates-visceral-fat-has-a-profoundly-negative-effect-on-cognitive-abilities-164382

Eske, J. (2023, January 6). *Leaky gut syndrome: What it is, symptoms, and treatments.* https://www.medicalnewstoday.com/articles/3 26117#summary

Food allergy versus food intolerance. (2019, March 15). Allergy Insider. https://www.thermofisher.com/allergy/wo/en /living-with-allergies/food-allergies/food- allergy-vs-food-intolerance.html

Food allergy (2021, December 31). Mayo Clinic. https://www.mayoclinic.org/diseases- conditions/food-allergy/symptoms-causes/syc- 20355095

Fluid retention (oedema). (2012). Better Health Channel. https://www.betterhealth.vic.gov.au/health/co nditionsandtreatments/Fluid-retention-oedema

Fulghum, D. (2007a, June 22). *How drinking fluids can help you manage constipation.* WebMD; WebMD. https://www.webmd.com/digestive- disorders/water-a-fluid-way-to-manage- constipation

Fulghum, D. (2007b, June 25). *Exercise to ease constipation.* WebMD. https://www.webmd.com/digestive- disorders/exercise-curing-constipation-via- movement

Gastroesophageal reflux disease (GERD) (2023, January 4). Mayo Clinic. https://www.mayoclinic.org/diseases- conditions/gerd/symptoms-causes/syc- 20361940

Godman, H. (2021, August 1). *Chronic gut inflammation: Coping with inflammatory bowel disease.* Harvard Health. https://www.health.harvard.edu/diseases-and-conditions/chronic-gut-inflammation-coping-with-inflammatory-bowel-disease

Gunnars, K. (2020, October 22). *22 high-fiber foods you should eat.* Healthline. https://www.healthline.com/nutrition/22-high-fiber-foods#faq

Gustafson, C. (2017). Bruce Lipton, Ph.D.: The jump from cell culture to consciousness. *Integrative Medicine (Encinitas, Calif.), 16*(6), 44–50. https://www.ncbi.nlm.nih.gov/pmc/articles/PMC6438088/

Haththotuwa, R. N., Wijeyaratne, C. N., & Senarath, U. (2020, January 1). *Chapter 1 - Worldwide epidemic of obesity* (T. A. Mahmood, S. Arulkumaran, & F. A. Chervenak, Eds.). ScienceDirect. https://www.sciencedirect.com/science/article/abs/pii/B9780128179215000011

Hill, M. (2018, November 16). *4 ways to improve your digestion if you're stressed.* Healthline. https://www.healthline.com/health/four-ways-to-improve-your-gut-if-youre-stressed

How high blood pressure can affect your body. (2022, January 14). Mayo Clinic. https://www.mayoclinic.org/diseases-conditions/high-blood-pressure/in-depth/high-blood-pressure/art-20045868

How salt can impact your blood pressure, heart, and kidneys. (2017, June 15). Cleveland Clinic. https://health.clevelandclinic.org/kidneys-salt-and-blood-pressure-you-need-a-delicate-balance/

How to properly combine foods to improve digestive health. (2018, October 25). LiveFit. https://livefitfood.ca/blogs/news/how-to-properly-combine-foods-in-order-to-improve-digestive-health

Incredible benefits of Himalayan salt. (2023, October 2) Healthy Human. https://healthyhumanlife.com/blogs/news/benefits-of-himalayan-salt

Irritable bowel syndrome. (n.d.). Mayo Clinic. https://www.mayoclinic.org/diseases-conditions/irritable-bowel-syndrome/symptoms-causes/syc-20360016

Irvine, U. of C. (2008, October 10). *How fatty foods curb hunger.* ScienceDaily. https://www.sciencedaily.com/releases/2008/10/081007123647.htm

Is a food intolerance making weight loss difficult? (2014, May 25). YorkTest. https://www.yorktest.com/us/blog/is-a-food-intolerance-making-it-difficult-for-you-to-lose-weight/

Is inflammation preventing you from losing weight? (n.d.). Dropbio Health.

https://www.dropbiohealth.com/health-resources/inflammation-weight-loss

Keys, A., Mienotti, A., Karvonen, M. j., Aravanis, C., Blackburn, H., Buzina, R., Djordjevic, B. S., Dontas, A. S., Fidanza, F., Keys, M. H., Kromhout, D., Nedeljkovic, S., Punsar, S., Seccareccia, F., & Toshima, H. (1986). The diet and 15-year death rate in the seven countries study. *American Journal of Epidemiology*, *124*(6), 903–915. https://doi.org/10.1093/oxfordjournals.aje.a114480

Lawler, M. (2018, August 31). *Celebs who love the keto diet: Kim Kardashian, Halle Berry, and more*. Everyday Health. https://www.everydayhealth.com/ketogenic-diet/diet/celebrities-cant-get-enough-ketogenic-diet/

Lee, C.-Y. S., Goldstein, S. E., Dik, B. J., & Rodas, J. M. (2020). Sources of social support and gender in perceived stress and individual adjustment among Latina/o college-attending emerging adults. *Cultural Diversity and Ethnic Minority Psychology*, *26*(1), 134–147. https://doi.org/10.1037/cdp0000279

Lemos, J. de. (2020, December 16). *Why belly fat is dangerous and how to control it*. UT Southwestern Medical Center. https://utswmed.org/medblog/belly-fat/

LeWine, H. E. (Ed.). (2020, March 25). *How much water should you drink?* Harvard Health. https://www.health.harvard.edu/staying-healthy/how-much-water-should-you-drink

Loy, B. D., O'Connor, P. J., & Dishman, R. K. (2013). The effect of a single bout of exercise on energy and fatigue states: a systematic review and meta-analysis. *Fatigue: Biomedicine, Health & Behavior*, *1*(4), 223–242. https://doi.org/10.1080/21641846.2013.84326 6

Ludwig, D. S. (2019). The ketogenic diet: Evidence for optimism but high-quality research needed. *The Journal of Nutrition*, *150*(6). https://doi.org/10.1093/jn/nxz308

Mackenzie, M. (2016, September 26). *What your poop can tell you about your belly fat.* Women's Health. https://www.womenshealthmag.com/weight-loss/a19904841/poop-reveals-about-belly-fat/

Madel, R. (2012, April 10). *Exercise as stress relief.* Healthline. https://www.healthline.com/health/heart-disease/exercise-stress-relief#Check-with-Your-Doctor

Mawer, R. (2019, December 15). *A ketogenic diet to lose weight and fight disease.* Healthline. https://www.healthline.com/nutrition/ketogen ic-diet-and-weight-loss#What-is-a-ketogenic-diet?

Mensah, G. A., Croft, J. B., & Giles, W. H. (2002). The heart, kidney, and brain as target organs in hypertension. *Cardiology Clinics*, *20*(2), 225–247. https://doi.org/10.1016/s0733-8651(02)00004-8

Meredith, G. R., Rakow, D. A., Eldermire, E. R. B., Madsen, C. G., Shelley, S. P., & Sachs, N. A. (2020). Minimum time dose in nature to positively impact the mental health of college-aged students, and how to measure it: A scoping review. *Frontiers in Psychology*, *10*(2942). https://doi.org/10.3389/fpsyg.2019.02942

Nall, R. (2018, August 17). *How to relieve gas: Easy methods and remedies*. Medical news today. https://www.medicalnewstoday.com/articles/314530

NewBeauty Editors. (2017, May 30). *The "salt depletion" diet this model does before photoshoots is actually really dangerous*. NewBeauty. https://www.newbeauty.com/how-models-prepare-for-photoshoot-salt-depletion

Nikolai Anitchkov, MD. (2006). University of Minnesota. http://www.epi.umn.edu/cvdepi/bio-sketch/anitchkov-nikolai

Nohe, M. (2020, January 22). *Celebrities with food allergies*. Allergy Amulet. https://www.allergyamulet.com/blog/celebrities-with-food-allergies

Obesity and overweight. (2021, June 9). World Health Organization. https://www.who.int/newsroom/fact-sheets/detail/obesity-and-overweight

Omega-3 fatty acids. (2019). Cleveland Clinic. https://my.clevelandclinic.org/health/articles/17290-omega-3-fatty-acids

Palinski-Wade, E. (2016, March 26). *Eat fat to reduce belly fat*. For Dummies. https://www.dummies.com/article/body-mind-spirit/physical-health-well-being/diet-nutrition/belly-fat-diet/eat-fat-to-reduce-belly-fat-169518/

Peng, A. W., Juraschek, S. P., Appel, L. J., Miller, E. R., & Mueller, N. T. (2019). Effects of the dash diet and sodium intake on bloating. *The American Journal of Gastroenterology*, *114*(7), 1109–1115. https://doi.org/10.14309/ajg.0000000000000283

Petre, A. (2017). *8 foods that can cause constipation*. Healthline. https://www.healthline.com/nutrition/8-foods-that-cause-constipation

Petre, A. (2020, January 31). *7 foods that can cause constipation*. Healthline. https://www.healthline.com/nutrition/8-foods-that-cause-constipation#3.-Processed-grains

Plowe, K. (2022, March 21). *4 reasons your weight-loss diet is making you gassy, and how to fix it*. Livestrong.com. https://www.livestrong.com/article/271843-why-do-i-have-gas-when-losing-weight

Proctor, L. (2014). The integrative human microbiome project: Dynamic analysis of microbiome-host omics profiles during periods of human health and disease. *Cell Host & Microbe*, *16*(3), 276–289. https://doi.org/10.1016/j.chom.2014.08.014

Ruggeri, C. (2016, November 24). *8 Popular foods are responsible for 90+ percent of food allergies.* Dr. Axe. https://draxe.com/health/food-allergy-alternatives/

Symptoms & causes of gas in the digestive tract. (2019, October). National Institute of Diabetes and Digestive and Kidney Diseases. https://www.niddk.nih.gov/health-information/digestive-diseases/gas-digestive-tract/symptoms-causes

Symptoms & causes of gas in the digestive tract. (2023, October 4). National Institute of Diabetes and Digestive and Kidney Diseases. https://www.niddk.nih.gov/health-information/digestive-diseases/gas-digestive-tract/symptoms-causes

Sachdev, P. (2023, February 26). *High blood pressure symptoms.* WebMD. https://www.webmd.com/hypertension-high-blood-pressure/hypertension-symptoms-high-blood-pressure

Salt and sodium. (2019, May 7). Harvard School of Public Health. https://www.hsph.harvard.edu/nutritionsource/salt-and-sodium/

Salty foods: How sodium affects your weight. (n.d.). Creekside Family Practice. https://www.creeksidefamilypractice.com/blog/salty-foods-how-sodium-affects-your-weight#

Samra, R. A. (2010). *Fats and Satiety* (J.-P. Montmayeur & J. le Coutre, Eds.). PubMed; CRC Press/Taylor & Francis. https://www.ncbi.nlm.nih.gov/books/NBK53550/

Saturated fat. (2021, November 1). American Heart Association. https://www.heart.org/en/healthy-living/healthy-eating/eat-smart/fats/saturated-fats

Smith, J. (2023, April 11). *How to lose water weight: 6 ways.* Medical News today. https://www.medicalnewstoday.com/articles/320603#ways-to-lose-water-weight

Sodium in your diet. (2020). U.S. Food and Drug Administration. https://www.fda.gov/food/nutrition-education-resources-materials/sodium-your-diet

Sodium in your diet use the nutrition facts label and reduce your intake. (2021). U.S. Food and Drug Administration. https://www.fda.gov/media/84261/download

Sodium intake and health. (2019). Centers for Disease Control and Prevention. https://www.cdc.gov/salt/index.htm

Sodium intake for adults and children. (2012). World Health Organization. https://apps.who.int/iris/bitstream/handle/10665/77985/9789241504836_eng.pdf

Solinas, C., Corpino, M., Maccioni, R., & Pelosi, U. (2010). Cow's milk protein allergy. *The Journal of Maternal-Fetal & Neonatal Medicine, 23*(sup3), 76–79. https://doi.org/10.3109/14767058.2010.51210 3

The power of flat tummy slogans: How they motivate and encourage people. (n.d.). Best Slogans. https://www.bestslogans.com/list-ideas-taglines/flat-tummy-slogans/

13 things diet experts won't tell you about weight loss. (2012, March 19). ABC News. https://abcnews.go.com/Health/diet-secrets-13-things-experts-weight-loss-good/story?id=15954615

Wade, M. (2015, July 29). *The risks of belly fat.* WebMD. https://www.webmd.com/obesity/features/tAhe-risks-of-belly-fat

Walker-Smith, J. A. (1988). Dietary protein intolerance. *Elsevier EBooks,* 144–184. https://doi.org/10.1016/b978-0-407-01320-9.50011-x

Walters, S. (2018, March 15). *Do you lose weight when you poop? Average weight of poop.* Healthline. https://www.healthline.com/health/do-you-lose-weight-when-you-poop

WebMD Editorial Contributors. (2015, September 24). *What kind of poop do I have?* WebMD. https://www.webmd.com/digestive-disorders/poop-chart-bristol-stool-scale

WebMD Contributors. (2022, November 7). *Testing for food allergies.* WebMD. https://www.webmd.com/allergies/food-allergy-test

WebMD Contributors. (2023, April 25). *Top exercises for belly fat.* WebMD. https://www.webmd.com/fitness-exercise/top-exercises-belly-fat

Wellness & Prevention. (2023, May 30). *Good fats vs. Bad fats.* Scripps Health. https://www.scripps.org/news_items/4359-good-fats-vs-bad-fats

Westphal, S. A. (2008). Obesity, abdominal obesity, and insulin resistance. *Clinical Cornerstone, 9*(1), 23–31. https://doi.org/10.1016/s1098-3597(08)60025-3

WHO Media Team. (2023, July 17). *WHO updates guidelines on fats and carbohydrates.* WHO. https://www.who.int/news/item/17-07-2023-who-updates-guidelines-on-fats-and-carbohydrates

Why beans make you fart and how to prevent it. (2023, April 18). Cleveland Clinic. https://health.clevelandclinic.org/why-do-beans-make-you-fart/

Winham, D. M., & Hutchins, A. M. (2011). Perceptions of flatulence from bean consumption among adults in 3 feeding studies. *Nutrition Journal*, *10*(1). https://doi.org/10.1186/1475-2891-10-128

Your digestive system & how it works. (2023a, May 11). National Institute of Diabetes and Digestive and Kidney Diseases. https://www.niddk.nih.gov/health-information/digestive-diseases/digestive-system-how-it-works

www.ingramcontent.com/pod-product-compliance
Lightning Source LLC
Chambersburg PA
CBHW022057020426
42335CB00012B/726